JOHANNES DE MIRFELD
of St Bartholomew's, Smithfield

JOHANNES DE MIRFELD

of St Bartholomew's, Smithfield

HIS LIFE AND WORKS

BY

SIR PERCIVAL HORTON-SMITH HARTLEY

C.V.O., M.A., M.D., F.R.C.P.

*Consulting Physician to St Bartholomew's Hospital
and to the Brompton Hospital
Sometime Fellow of St John's College, Cambridge*

AND

HAROLD RICHARD ALDRIDGE

M.A.

*Formerly Scholar of Peterhouse, Cambridge
Assistant Keeper in the Department of Manuscripts
in the British Museum*

CAMBRIDGE

AT THE UNIVERSITY PRESS

1936

CAMBRIDGE UNIVERSITY PRESS
Cambridge, New York, Melbourne, Madrid, Cape Town,
Singapore, São Paulo, Delhi, Mexico City

Cambridge University Press
The Edinburgh Building, Cambridge CB2 8RU, UK

Published in the United States of America by Cambridge University Press, New York

www.cambridge.org
Information on this title: www.cambridge.org/9781107686052

© Cambridge University Press 1936

This publication is in copyright. Subject to statutory exception
and to the provisions of relevant collective licensing agreements,
no reproduction of any part may take place without the written
permission of Cambridge University Press.

First published 1936
First paperback edition 2013

A catalogue record for this publication is available from the British Library

ISBN 978-1-107-68605-2 Paperback

Cambridge University Press has no responsibility for the persistence or
accuracy of URLs for external or third-party internet websites referred to in
this publication, and does not guarantee that any content on such websites is,
or will remain, accurate or appropriate.

PREFACE

THE work, which we now present, dealing with the first writings of a medical nature known to be associated with any English Hospital, had its origin in the following manner.

The writings of the late Sir Norman Moore had familiarised all connected with St Bartholomew's with the fact that in the latter half of the fourteenth century, in the days of Richard II, there lived and wrote within the Priory of St Bartholomew in Smithfield a certain Johannes de Mirfeld, or, in its English rendering, John Mirfeld (or Mirfield).

Who exactly he was, whether a physician connected with St Bartholomew's, layman or cleric, and if the latter, whether a full Canon of the Augustinian Order, was not clear, for much had been postulated categorically concerning him which has now been proved to be incorrect.

It has also been known since 1869, from the researches of A. J. Horwood, that this John Mirfeld was the author of a book, entitled the *Florarium Bartholomei*. This work is a lengthy theological treatise, the only MSS. thereof, so far as was then known, being in the Libraries of the British Museum and of Gray's Inn. In addition to the purely theological chapters, however, the MS. contains one medical chapter, entitled "De Medicis et eorum Medicinis".

In the Library of the British Museum there is to be found another lengthy MS., a medical work, entitled the *Breviarium Bartholomei*, a copy of which also exists in the Library of Pembroke College, Oxford. Riley had shown in 1877 that this work was also written by a John Mirfeld, a resident in the Monastery of St Bartholomew in Smithfield. The discovery by Sir Norman Moore of an acrostic in the *Breviarium* similar to the one already shown by

Horwood to exist in the *Florarium*, proved the identity of authorship, and demonstrated that both works should be attributed to the same John Mirfeld.

In his Fitz-Patrick Lectures on *The History of the Study of Medicine in the British Isles* (1908) Sir Norman Moore referred at some length to John Mirfeld and his writings. Nevertheless, but little was known about his life; and his MSS. have never been translated, though his work has been well known since the publication in 1882 of a small section entitled "Sinonoma Bartholomei". This is to be found only in the Oxford MS. of the *Breviarium*, and is in fact a dictionary or glossary of medical terms employed in the *Breviarium* itself. It has been quoted in the *New English Dictionary*, owing to some of its definitions being in English, and has led, as will be shown, to the placing of a disproportionate value upon Mirfeld's writings.

Bearing in mind the interest which his works—dating from the fourteenth century, and being the earliest medical writings associated with St Bartholomew's—naturally possess for all who are connected with that famous Foundation, it seemed desirable that some attempt at translation should be made, and some effort to elucidate further the life-story of the Author, who had been acclaimed as one of the earliest physicians associated with its activities.

A preliminary examination of the MSS. in the British Museum made it clear that, if only from their size and voluminous contents, a full translation would be a task of great magnitude. We have calculated, indeed, that the printing of the Latin text of the *Breviarium* alone would fill a volume of 2400 pages of a size similar to that used in the present publication. In consequence, it was decided to translate certain chapters and extracts only, which would give those interested some idea of the character of the works. From the *Breviarium* the following portions have been finally chosen:

The *Proemium or Introduction*.

The chapter on *The Signs of Death* (with the additions contained in the Lambeth Palace MS.), and also that on *Consumption*, the latter subject possessing a special interest for the editors of this work. Short extracts then follow, giving formulae for the making of *Gun Powder*, the prescription for the *Emplastrum Bartholomei* and a note on *Weights and Measures*, this section being concluded by the *Epilogue* to the work.

As regards the *Florarium*, the *Proemium* thereto has been translated, then follows the chapter "De Medicis et Eorum Medicinis" and finally the *Epilogue*.

Appendices, giving details of the MSS. used, and abstracts of numerous legal documents referred to in the text, conclude the work.

As regards the preparation of the text, examination of the MSS. showed that they were written in the monastic Latin of the day, with arbitrary punctuation and division into paragraphs, and in the abbreviated script (as exemplified in Plates I–III) current at the end of the fourteenth century. It was at once evident that no text, if it was to be of any value, could be prepared without expert assistance. Very fortunately Mr H. R. Aldridge, late Scholar of Peterhouse, Cambridge, and now Assistant Keeper in the Department of Manuscripts at the British Museum, was interested in the subject, and with his invaluable and untiring help the work has been carried out, the spare time of several years being devoted to this purpose.

With reference to the *Breviarium* the texts of the two known MSS., those in the British Museum and in the Library of Pembroke College, Oxford, have been collated, and a satisfactory text produced. In the case of the *Florarium*, the task proved more difficult. The only manuscript of this work mentioned by Sir Norman Moore, viz. the one in the British Museum, proved very corrupt.

Mr Aldridge has however succeeded in tracing five other
manuscripts, details of which are given in Appendix B,
and by their collation—for not one is perfectly reliable—a
reasonable text has been obtained. This medieval Latin
rendering and its English translation are to be found set
forth on opposite pages in the body of the work.

In his writings, portions of which are thus set forth,
John Mirfeld shows himself as a kindly man, who, in his
chamber in the Priory, wrote his two treatises for the
benefit of his fellow-men: the *Florarium*—a flower-garden
of divine beauty—to guide them along the strait and nar-
row path leading to salvation: the *Breviarium* to provide
them with a work, from which they could cull with ease the
remedies found useful in those early days in the treatment
of the many ills referred to.

His writings upon examination now prove to be entirely
medieval, entirely scholastic, and to contain no original
work, and are thus in a sense disappointing. The description
of the various maladies referred to, and the remedies ad-
vised, are based only on *Authority*: the well-known classical
and medieval writers, as will be seen in the text, being
quoted at length, and often verbatim. Mingled with this
veneration for Authority are not a few *Charms*, recalling the
Anglo-Saxon Leechdoms, and some examples of pure *Magic*.
Of more value from the modern point of view are the
sensible remarks on the value of exercise in the medical
chapter in the *Florarium*, which possess almost a modern
ring, though they prove to be direct quotations from
Bernardus de Gordonio.

Nevertheless, Mirfeld's writings possess an interest of
their own, as showing from works written in the Priory—
which was responsible to some extent for the well-ordering
of the Hospital—what was the state of medical knowledge
in London some five centuries ago, at a time when, we
may recall, the Hospital itself was no longer young, but

had already been carrying out its beneficent work for nearly three hundred years. The chapter on consumption also has a pathetic interest of its own, for if it be true—as is commonly believed—that the great national hero, Edward, the Black Prince, himself died of this disease, then this chapter gives probably some indication of the lines of treatment which were actually followed in his individual case.

As regards the life-history of our Author, but little was previously known about him beyond the fact that he lived and wrote his works within the Priory in Smithfield, towards the end of the fourteenth century. Mr Aldridge has made extensive and laborious researches in all likely places, in order to discover, if possible, further information in regard to him, and has met with a considerable measure of success, the details of which are given in the text. In particular it will be shown that John Mirfeld (or Mirfield) was connected with the great Yorkshire family of that name, that he came to London, resided in the Priory, and afterwards took the Tonsure, and after passing through the various minor orders, was finally ordained Priest in London on the 10th of April 1395. It seems clear that though a Cleric, and residing in the Priory, he never joined the Monastic Order and never became an Augustinian Canon, but remained a simple Capellanus or Chaplain, an unbeneficed Priest. His exact connection with the Hospital of St Bartholomew must remain doubtful, though it may be that he acted as one of the Hospital Chaplains. The idea that he studied at Oxford, and attended the medical lectures of Nicholas Tyngewich (Physician to Edward I) in that University is based, we believe, on a misinterpretation of a passage in the text of the *Breviarium*. He was, however, in any case a man of wide reading and fully conversant, as will be seen, with all the medical writings of his predecessors, upon which a physician in those days was expected to base his knowledge.

He was evidently further a man of considerable business capacity and well trusted by his friends, as the various documents to be quoted, giving some idea of his trusteeships, indicate. As we have already hinted, his kindly thought for others is manifested in his writings.

He died, as we shall show, in 1407; his will, a copy of which we reproduce, being dated the 15th of April, and proved on the 5th of May in that year in the Court of the Archdeacon of London. In it he gives instructions that he is to be buried in the Church of St Botolph, without Aldersgate, and presumably he was there interred.

From what has been said, it will be apparent that the chief labour involved in the preparation of this work must, of necessity, have fallen upon the shoulders of Mr Aldridge. It is he who has searched the records, discovered fresh texts, collated the various manuscripts, and prepared from the medieval script the Latin texts, as finally printed. My easier task has been to initiate the work, to help it forward at every juncture, and to collaborate in the translation of the text, and in the preparation of the various introductions. Should the work prove acceptable to those to whom it is dedicated, those who have an affection for the famous twin foundations of Rahere, the Priory and the Hospital of St Bartholomew, to Mr Aldridge must the chief credit be given.

In conclusion it is our pleasant duty to tender our grateful thanks to those who in so many ways have helped us in our work. To His Grace the Archbishop of Canterbury and his Librarians at Lambeth, as also to the President and Court of Governors of Sion College, our thanks are due for permission to remove the MSS. of the *Florarium*, in their possession, to the British Museum, for closer study. To the Librarians of Sion College our thanks are also rendered for their courtesy, during the study of the manuscript in that Institution.

We are grateful also to the Treasurer and Masters of the

Bench of the Honourable Society of Gray's Inn, and to Mr Severn, their Librarian, and his Assistants, for their courtesy in permitting us to consult the copy of the *Florarium* in their possession.

To Prof. R. G. Collingwood, M.A., F.B.A., till lately Fellow and Librarian of Pembroke College, Oxford, we are especially indebted for his consideration and kindness in permitting us to study the manuscript of the *Breviarium* belonging to the College, both in his own rooms and in the Bodleian, usually at short notice and sometimes at considerable personal inconvenience to himself. Our thanks are also due to Bodley's Librarian and the Librarian of the University of Cambridge for the facilities which they have afforded us.

To Dr Arnold Chaplin, the learned Harveian Librarian of the Royal College of Physicians, to Dr G. G. Coulton, to Prof. G. E. Gask, F.R.C.S., Mr L. G. H. Horton-Smith, Canon C. W. Foster, D.Litt., the Rev. Hugh P. Jones, the Rev. C. G. Challenger, to Mr Fulton of the Oriental Department and to several colleagues on the Staff of the Department of Manuscripts at the British Museum, and many other learned friends—to whom enquiries have been addressed, and who have always responded with unfailing and helpful regularity—we tender our grateful thanks.

To Sir D'Arcy Power, K.B.E., F.R.C.S., and to Prof. Charles Singer, M.D., we offer a special meed of gratitude for their ready kindness in reading our manuscripts and for much helpful advice, and many valuable suggestions.

Lastly, we should like to thank the officials of the University Press for the care and trouble which they have taken in the printing and production of this work.

PERCIVAL HORTON-SMITH HARTLEY

February, 1936

CONTENTS

Preface   *page* vii

I. INTRODUCTION   1
    I. The Life of Johannes de Mirfeld   3
    II. Johannes de Mirfeld as a Medical Writer   25

II. THE *BREVIARIUM BARTHOLOMEI*   35
    I. Introductory Remarks   36
    II. *Proemium*, Latin   46
        English Translation   47
    III. *De Signis Malis*, Latin   54
        English Translation   55
    IV. Chapter: *De Ptisi*, Latin   74
        English Translation   75
    Other Extracts

    V. *Pulvis pro instrumento bellico* (Gunpowder)
        Latin   90
        English Translation   91
    VI. *Emplastrum Bartholomei*
        Latin   90
        English Translation   91
    VII. *De Ponderibus et Mensuris*
        Latin   92
        English Translation   93
    VIII. Epilogue, Latin   94
        English Translation   95

page

III. THE *FLORARIUM BARTHOLOMEI* 97

  I. Introductory Remarks 98

  II. *Proemium*, Latin 114
    English Translation 115

  III. Chapter: *De Medicis et Eorum Medicinis*
    Latin 122
    English Translation 123

  IV. Epilogue, Latin 160
    English Translation 161

APPENDICES

  A. Notes on the MSS. used for the text of the
    Breviarium Bartholomei 167

  B. Notes on the MSS. used for the text of
    the *Florarium Bartholomei* 169

  C. Abstracts from Deeds and Documents
    referred to in the Text 175

PLATES

I. *Breviarium Bartholomei*   *to face page* 54
    Beginning of Chapter *De Signis Malis*

II. *Breviarium Bartholomei*
    First portion of Chapter *De Ptisi*   ,,   74

III. *Breviarium Bartholomei*
    Second and concluding portion of the chapter
    De Ptisi   ,,   88

IV. Will of Johannes de Mirfeld   ,,   176

§ I

Introduction

I

INTRODUCTION

JOHANNES DE MIRFELD, author of the *Breviarium Bartholomei*, had already been advanced to an honourable place amidst medieval English medical writers, both by the publication of a small section of this work—the *Sinonoma* or Glossary[1]—as well as by the labours of eminent bibliographers, when the late Sir Norman Moore, in the first of his Fitz-Patrick Lectures for 1905–1906,[2] devoted considerable attention not only to this book but also to another work by the same author, namely, the *Florarium Bartholomei*.

In the course of his lecture Sir Norman mentioned that Mirfeld was the first genuine writer on Medicine to be in any way connected with St Bartholomew's Hospital as distinct from the chronicler of the miraculous cures recorded in the *Book of the Foundation*.[3] For this reason alone it is to be hoped that the publication of these additional extracts from Mirfeld's works may be held justified, even though an examination should disclose the fact that they do not contain anything that can be regarded as an original contribution to medical science in itself, or new to the student of medical history.

The value indeed of these excerpts lies rather in the fact that they provide the modern reader with a genuine historical document: a record which demonstrates the nature

[1] The *Sinonoma*, or Glossary of medical terms, the meanings of which are given sometimes in Latin and sometimes in English (edited by J. L. G. Mowat, M.A., in *Anecdota Oxoniensia*, Mediaeval and Modern Series, Vol. I, Part I, 1882). It is one of the authorities quoted in the *New English Dictionary*.
[2] *On the History of the Study of Medicine in the British Isles* (Oxford, Clarendon Press, 1908), p. 44.
[3] British Museum MS. Vespasian B IX; see also St Bartholomew's Hospital Reports, Vol. XXI.

of the medical doctrines accepted by an author who was a contemporary both of the Black Prince and of Chaucer, and an acquaintance, if not a friend, of Adam Rous, surgeon to King Edward III; who would seem to have lived for many years within the Priory and to have been closely connected with the Hospital of St Bartholomew in Smithfield; and who may actually have been within the precincts at the very moment when Wat Tyler was brought in to die after that eventful interview with the young king under the conventual walls which provides the most picturesque, as well as the most decisive, incident of the Peasants' Revolt of A.D. 1381.

Before, however, embarking upon any discussion as to the nature of his works, it will be advisable to state the little that can be ascertained definitely concerning the writer himself.

I. THE LIFE OF JOHANNES DE MIRFELD

Johannes de Mirfeld has generally been described as a Canon of the Augustinian Priory of St Bartholomew, Smithfield. Such an assertion, however, is unfounded: for a study of available records clearly demonstrates that Mirfeld was never admitted to full membership of the Augustinian Order, although he appears to have resided for many years within the precincts of one of its Houses, and gave to his books the name of the Institution with which he was thus associated.

That he was in fact not a full Canon can be readily deduced from an inspection of the Clerical Subsidy Roll for A.D. 1379,[1] where it will be found that "Johannes Meryfeld" is described not as a Canon ("Canonicus"), but as one of the "Clerks of the Priory" ("Clerici eiusdem Prioratus") of St Bartholomew Smithfield: and that he

---

[1] Now preserved in the Public Record Office. See the extract from it relating to St Bartholomew's Priory printed by E. A. Webb, *The Records of St Bartholomew's Priory... West Smithfield* (1921), Vol. I, p. 172.

paid, as his share of the tax, no more than 4*d.*, whereas each Canon was assessed at not less than 3*s.* 4*d.*[1]

Moreover, the name of John Mirfeld does not appear in the Register of Bishop Braybroke as one of the Canons who voted at the election of Prior William Gedeney, an event which took place in 1382 whilst Mirfeld presumably was residing in the Priory.

Nor indeed would it appear from documents still extant that our author was ever known to his contemporaries as an Augustinian Canon. He was certainly not so regarded in 1395 by the Bishop who ordained him priest (and by whom he was enrolled simply as "ciuitatis Londonie"[2]), nor to the executrix who proved his will (who is called his mother) and who described him as a "Dominus" and "Capellanus", i.e. a fully ordained but unbeneficed priest who acted as a chaplain: had he been a Canon the records in each of these cases could hardly have failed to give such information. Again, Mirfeld when recording his various legal transactions never refers to himself by any style which implies membership of a monastic Order.[3]

It is impossible to state with precision the exact nature of his connection with the Priory and the Hospital of St Bartholomew, especially as the two institutions were distinct, though connected, and were quarrelling with each other during the earlier years of his residence in the Close to such an extent that the arbitration of the Bishop of London (Simon of Sudbury) became necessary.

All that has hitherto been discovered regarding this connection—in addition to the information obtained from the

[1] Not 30*s.* 4*d.* as given by E. A. Webb, *op. cit.*
[2] See Appendix C, p. 175.
[3] Mowat's statement that in 1392 and 1393 Mirfeld represented the Priory in the King's court (and the inference drawn therefrom that he was a senior Canon), is based upon a misinterpretation of certain entries in the *Calendarium Inquisitionum Post Mortem*, Vol. III (Record Commission, 1821). These entries merely relate to his conveyances of real property to the Priory.

Clerical Subsidy Roll previously mentioned—is an entry on the Patent Rolls dated the 4th of April 1390, which consists of a Royal Inspeximus and Confirmation of an Indenture between John de Mirfeld of the one part and the Prior (Thomas de Watford) and "Convent" of St Bartholomew of the other part. This enrolled agreement was dated the 9th of May 1362, and by its terms the Prior and Convent grant to Mirfeld an annual pension of 4*l.* 8*s.* for life, with the stipulation that if this pension be not paid, then Mirfeld (or his attorney) shall have power to obtain an equivalent amount of food and drink in lieu thereof, by levying, if necessary, a distress upon the Priory's possessions in London; furthermore, the Priory leases to Mirfeld, at an annual rent of 4*s.*, "a certain chamber...on the South side of the said Church, and adjoining the Great Altar", which chamber Sir Norman Moore identified as the room formerly situated at the level of the triforium and built out into the Close from the South wall of the Priory Church at a spot corresponding roughly to the second bay eastward of that which now contains Prior Bolton's window.

One feature of this deed which appears to have been generally overlooked is that whilst, according to the contract which it embodies, the Priory is given no power to terminate the lease of the chamber, yet Mirfeld is permitted to retain possession of his room for so long as he shall think fit, and may vacate it at any time upon giving three months' notice.[1] It is difficult to believe that such terms would have been granted, or such latitude permitted, to a man who had accepted the conditions imposed upon those who became full members of the Augustinian Order; and this provides yet another indication that Mirfeld's position in the Priory was that of a resident stranger—a "commorans"

---

[1] "...quamdiu eam tenere voluerit et in casu quo eam amplius tenere noluerit premuniet predictos priorem et conuentum per vnum quartum anni."

(or "sojourner") as he is termed in the *Incipit* of the Oxford copy of the *Breviarium Bartholomei*—rather than that of a member of the Order.[1]

In the absence of other evidence it would normally follow that the annuity was given in return either for personal services rendered to the monastery, or else for some substantial gift (generally of land) made either by the annuitant himself or by some person acting on his behalf. Into the latter category, however, Mirfeld's various donations to the Priory do not seem to fall; for, as will be shown later, the various properties which he transferred to St Bartholomew's were probably not his own private possessions but those which he held merely as trustee for others. Nor is there any record extant to show that the corrody was originally granted by royal command. These facts, taken in conjunction with the entry in the Clerical Subsidy Roll, seem to justify the assumption that Mirfeld's position in the Priory was that of a salaried official, although it is impossible to be certain of the actual nature of the services which he performed.

No evidence is available to explain why the Inspeximus was obtained, but it is just possible that Mirfeld was contemplating ordination, and that he desired either to resign his duties in the Priory, or to transfer to the Hospital, but still to retain the lease of his chamber, and that he therefore went to the trouble of obtaining the royal recognition of the deed executed nearly thirty years before. On the other hand it is quite possible that an attempt was being made by royal officials to obtain a corrody from the Priory, and that Mirfeld was forced to secure his Inspeximus in order to protect his interests from being overridden.

With the exception of the grants made by him to the Priory of St Bartholomew (and to which reference will

[1] *Infra*, p. 39.

again be made), no further information of an authentic nature has hitherto been discovered concerning Mirfeld. He has usually been regarded as an Augustinian Canon, but sometimes, however, as a layman who was a professional physician. The following facts, now brought to light, may perhaps have the effect of modifying these views.

The Register of Robert de Braybroke, Bishop of London from 1381 to 1404, contains a section (curiously neglected by the historians of St Bartholomew's) in which are recorded the names of those who were ordained to the priesthood either by the Bishop himself or by his deputies. A search of these ordination lists discloses the fact that on Saturday, the 19th of September 1394, one John Mirfeld, of the City of London ("Johannes Mirfeld, Ciuitatis Londonie"[1]), presented himself in St Paul's Cathedral amongst the candidates for admission to the order of Acolyte, but for some reason now unknown he was refused ordination. The cryptic note written against his name, "iste non fuit ordinatus" ("this man was not ordained"), gives no indication as to the cause of his rejection. Probably he merely lacked a "title", because his pension was too meagre to be considered as sufficient for the purpose; but one is tempted to suggest that, since he had already written a medical book,[2] he was regarded as a physician and one who might, it was feared, have incurred such an "irregularity" during his practice as to be disqualified for the higher orders of the priesthood—a problem which he himself discusses at length in the Florarium. Whatever may have been the impediment to his promotion, it did not, however, prove permanent; for at a subsequent ordination, held in St Paul's on Saturday, the 6th of March following (1395), all was well, and he was made first an Acolyte, and then a Sub-

[1] See Appendix C, p. 175.
[2] The *Breviarium* was probably composed between 1380 and 1395 (see p. 38).

deacon. Here an interesting fact emerges. His title is set down as being "The Master and Confraternity of the Hospital of St Bartholomew, Smithfield" ("...Magistri et Confraternitatis Hospitalis Sancti Bartholomei in Smethefeld Londonie"), which proves that he was to derive his subsistence, not from the Priory, but from the Hospital, since the former is designated in the register as the "Prior and Convent". Mirfeld is not described as a "Canon" of the Priory, nor is he called a "Brother" of the Hospital; and it is difficult to ascertain his exact status, since he is simply set down as being "of the diocese of London". He proceeded normally to the Diaconate on the 27th of March and finally was ordained a Priest on Saturday the 10th of April 1395, still retaining the "Hospital" as his title.[1]

Nothing further is heard of him until his death, which must have occurred between the 15th of April (xvii Kalends of May) and the 5th (iii Nones) of May 1407, since his will was made on the first, and proved in the Archdeaconry Court of London on the second, of these two dates.[2] In this will (which was a nuncupative, i.e. an unwritten, or verbal, one) he described himself as a "Dominus" and a "Capellanus" or Chaplain; in other words, he was an unbeneficed priest. He directed that he should be buried, not within the Priory of St Bartholomew as would be expected were he a Canon, but in the cemetery of St Botolph, without Aldersgate, which at the time of his death was the parish church of the inhabitants of St Bartholomew's Close. He bequeathed all his possessions to "Margaret Schadelok", whom he named sole executrix and described as his mother. The actual identity of this Margaret is a mystery, for all the efforts which we have made to glean further information about her have proved fruitless: nor has her discovery provided any other clues

[1] See Appendix C, p. 175.   [2] See Appendix C, p. 176.

concerning the ancestry or mode of life of her son, and these must now be sought elsewhere.

Accordingly, the following abstract of a deed, executed in London on the 1st of April 1379 and copied into the Hustings Rolls now preserved among the archives at the Guildhall of the Corporation of the City of London, merits consideration:[1]

KNOW ALL MEN, etc...., that I, John Mirfeld, have granted...to John Herthull, "clerk", all those tenements, etc., situate in the parish of St. Andrew, Holborn, which lately came to me and to William atte Vyne, citizen of London, by the deaths of Dom. William de Mirfeld and Dom. Roger de Barnesburgh, Clerks (they having obtained them by feoffment of Elias de Sutton, Clerk), and which the said William atte Vyne has already released to me; To be held by the aforesaid John Herthull for life, with remainder to Master Adam Rous, Surgeon ("surrigicus") to the Lord King, and to his heirs for ever. I grant also to the same John Herthull all those tenements situate in the parishes of "St. Mildrithe in Pulletria" [St Mildred in the Poultry] and St. Edmund the King in Lombard Street, and in "Bercherneslane" [Birchin Lane], of which I, together with William atte Vyne and Robert Bryen, received joint possession lately by the gift of Adam Rous and which the said William and Robert have already released to me; To be held by the aforesaid John Herthull for life, with remainder to the said Adam Rous and his heirs. Dated, London, 1st of April, 2 Richard II [1379].

Professor George E. Gask has shown[2] that Adam Rous was appointed Surgeon to King Edward III between the years 1349 and 1359 and that his will (which was proved on the 25th of July 1379)[3] was executed on the 27th of April 1379, that is within less than a month after the date of the deed quoted above. In this will Adam Rous bequeathed to the Prior and Convent of St Bartholomew de Westsmythe-feld the reversions of certain tenements and rents held by John Herthull, clerk, in the parishes of St Andrew de Hol-

---

[1] Hustings Roll 107, No. 135. See Appendix C, p. 177.
[2] In his paper entitled "The Medical Staff of King Edward III", printed in *Proceedings of the Royal Society of Medicine*, Vol. XIX, No. 1, 1926, p. 1.
[3] Hustings Roll 108, No. 13.

bourn, St Mildred, St Edmund the King in Lumbardestrete, Bercherneslane, and All Hallows the Great in the Ropery. The various properties comprising this legacy (with the exception of those situated in the parish of All Hallows) are obviously identifiable as the subject-matter of the conveyance to Herthull quoted above, and which (excluding the tenements obtained from William de Mirfeld and Roger de Barnesburgh in St Andrew's) Rous had previously given to John Mirfeld and his two co-feoffees Robert Brien and William atte Vyne,[1] probably upon condition that they should ultimately be conveyed to Herthull or to some other person whom Rous should stipulate.[2]

It would seem then that Mirfeld was evidently acting in a fiduciary capacity on behalf of Adam Rous, with whom he must obviously have been on terms at least of business acquaintanceship, even if not of personal friendship; and it may well be that the man to whom Mirfeld refers in the *Breviarium* as "My Master" was none other than the Royal Surgeon himself; that is, indeed, if the "Master" had any existence in reality and was not, as appears more probable, merely a literary abstraction. Reference to this problem will be made below (pp. 22, 23).

[1] The grant of the houses in St Mildred's was dated 11 December, 1 Richard II [1377] and can be found in Hustings Roll 106, No. 74. The deed states that King Edward III granted the property to Rous for life by Letters Patent, dated 4 Nov. 1361; and in fee, by a further patent, dated 1 Sept. 1372. (N.B. These two patents have been printed in abstract by Prof. Gask, *op. cit.*) The property formed the subject of a law-suit between Rous and the Priory in 1362.

That granted in St Edmund the King, Lombard Street, and Berchernes-lane is registered in Hustings Roll 107, No. 11, and is dated 19 July, 2 Richard II [1378].

[2] These complex transactions arose owing to the fact that the law at that date prevented a man from making a grant of land to, or a settlement upon, himself: in order to found a trust which should operate after his death, it was necessary for him to convey to a friend, who would re-convey to the trustees (including perhaps the "settlor"). By associating several friends as joint trustees, the settlor obtained the advantages of the doctrine of survivorship, thus avoiding payment of dues to his feudal lord on his own death: the surviving trustee formed another trust in the same way, thus continuing the process. (N.B. The foregoing applies to William de Mirfeld as well as to Rous.)

It is with the *William de Mirfeld*, mentioned above in John's deed, that we are now more chiefly concerned, since upon him depends the sole clue to the family and status of our author.

The important family of Mirfeld, which derived its name from Mirfield in Yorkshire, rose during the fourteenth and fifteenth centuries to a prominent position in the West Riding, built its own Chantry Chapel in Batley Church,[1] intermarried with the most influential local families, and supplied some of the trusted "Conservators of the Peace".[2] A cadet of this house, the William de Mirfeld mentioned in John's deed, seems to have taken Orders, and then, in common with many of his contemporaries, to have sought his fortune in the service of the State, rather than in that of the Church. He entered the Royal Chancery during a most interesting period of its history and when it was still the great administrative department of the Government. He first appears there as a "king's clerk"[3] in the year 1342, and he eventually rose to the honourable position of a "Great Clerk", which corresponded in status to the modern Permanent Under-Secretaryship of State. In 1362 he became the Receiver of the Petitions presented in Parliament, and just about this time he also entered the service of the King's son, John of Gaunt, Duke of Lancaster, to whom he became a faithful Chief Attorney.[4] So well was he

[1] For further information about the family, see T. D. Whitaker, *Loidis and Elmete* (1816); and M. Sheard, *Records of the Parish of Batley* (1894).
[2] E.g., the Sir William de Mirfeld, Knight, whose name occurs in Appendix C, pp. 180, 181: he must not be confused with his namesake the Canon of Lincoln.
[3] *Calendar of Patent Rolls*, 1340–1343, pp. 494, 495. The King had presented his clerk William de Mirifeld to the living of Stoke by Nayland in Suffolk, but the Bishop of Norwich had admitted another. On the 8th of July 1342 the King pardoned the bishop and issued a mandate to the Justices of the Common Pleas to stay the process against the bishop for the non-admission of W. de Myrfeld. (The two different spellings of the name Mirfeld are noteworthy.)
[4] See *John of Gaunt's Register*, edited by Sir Sydney Armitage-Smith (Historical Society of Great Britain, 1911).

esteemed by his official superiors that in March 1371 he was appointed one of the four Commissioners to whom was entrusted the custody of the Great Seal during the absence from London of the recently appointed Chancellor Sir Robert de Thorpe.[1] He held a succession of livings, and on the 25th of November 1363 became Prebendary of Stow in Lindsey in the diocese of Lincoln: and at his death, which occurred on the 25th of July 1375 (possibly of the plague) he was the incumbent of Bradford in Yorkshire. Our researches have disclosed the fact that he made a will which was proved before the Official of the Archdeacon of London; and if a copy of this document could be recovered, much that is now obscure concerning John de Mirfeld would probably be made clear; but unfortunately the official register into which this will was transcribed has been destroyed with the exception of the index containing William de Mirfeld's name.[2] Apparently, William was buried in St Bartholomew's Priory; for the Roger de Barnesburgh mentioned above in John de Mirfeld's deed followed William to the grave shortly afterwards, and directed in his will,[3] which was dated the 4th of August 1375 and proved on the 16th of October (xvii Kalends of November) following, that should he happen to die in London, then he was to be buried in St Bartholomew's, Smithfield, and the Prior and Convent were to have twenty marks if they would make a "special mention" for his soul in the Masses celebrated for Dom. William de Mirfeld. This Roger de Barnesburgh was William de Mirfeld's colleague in the Chancery; he was his friend and apparently also his exe-

---

[1] E. Foss, *The Judges of England* (1851), Vol. iii, p. 466, gives the date as the 18th of March, which appears to be a mistake for the 28th. Thorpe was sworn on the 26th (*Calendar of Close Rolls*, 1369–1374, p. 287).

[2] It is now in the Principal Probate Registry, Somerset House (see Appendix C, p. 180). No copy of the will exists at Lincoln, where Canon C. W. Foster, M.A., D.Litt., most kindly assisted the editors by searching the Cathedral archives in an endeavour to trace it.

[3] For extracts therefrom see Appendix C, p. 181.

cutor and may even have been a distant kinsman owing to the marriage of relatives of both men into the Dodworth family. Roger names as the first of his executors his Chancery colleague the Elias de Sutton mentioned in the deed quoted above, and as the second a certain John de Conewyk de Herthull who may possibly be the John Herthull[1] to whom John de Mirfeld made his grant.

The premises in the parish of St Andrew Holborn which fell into the possession of John de Mirfeld during the year 1375 consisted originally of a series of houses, shops, and gardens which had been so combined together as to form three distinct properties possessing frontages on the south side of the royal highway of Holborn itself. Two of these were adjacent to each other and were separated from the third by a messuage belonging to St Bartholomew's Hospital which bounded them on the east. This separate and most easterly tenement, together with that on the extreme west, was owned by Barnesburgh and Sutton in partnership; whilst that lying adjacent to the Hospital property belonged to William de Mirfeld, and was perhaps the house in which he dwelt and to which reference was made during the proceedings of a Parliament which met in 1376, the year after his death.[2] William de Mirfeld seems to have wished to acquire all these properties and to make a disposition of them which should operate eventually to vest the whole of his interest in John de Mirfeld, though whether John was to take it on trust or as a gift is not quite clear. William accordingly obtained the co-operation of Barnesburgh and Sutton. The deeds relating to these transactions were copied into the Hustings Rolls,[3] from whence it appears that on the 23rd of July 1373 Sutton vested the two

[1] This name may possibly be a variant of, and derived from, Harthill in Yorkshire.
[2] "...en Holbourne en mesme l'Ostiel ou Sr William Mirfeld soleit demurer" (Rotuli Parliamentorum, Vol. II, p. 340).
[3] See Appendix C, pp. 178, 179.

most easterly properties in William de Mirfeld for life, with
the remainder after his death to John Mirfeld and William
atte Vyne jointly: and that on the same day, moreover, he
vested the most westerly set of premises in William de Mirfeld and Roger de Barnesburgh jointly for their lives, with
remainder after their deaths to John Mirfeld and William
atte Vyne. As a result of these grants, at the end of the year
1375 when William de Mirfeld and Barnesburgh were
both dead, all three properties belonged jointly to John de
Mirfeld and William atte Vyne. As has been seen, William
atte Vyne resigned his claims upon them,[1] and John Mirfeld granted them to John Herthull for life; and then in
1392, John Mirfeld and Robert Brian, acting perhaps instead of Herthull on behalf of the deceased Adam Rous,
conveyed them to St Bartholomew's Priory,[2] in whose possession they remained until the Dissolution. Finally, on the
14th of September 1543 they formed part of the property
which passed by a royal grant into the hands of Thomas
Berthelet the printer, from whom the site derived its
modern name of Bartlett's Buildings.[3]

In addition to this London property, William de Mirfeld
was found at his death to be possessed of the manors of
Fersley (in Calverley) and Shelf (in Halifax) in Yorkshire,
which he held "in chief" of the King, and had purchased
from Benedict de Normanton, his royal licence to do this
being dated the 4th of July 1348.[4] William de Mirfeld's
heirs[5] were his sister Joan (who died in 1380 leaving four

---

[1] Perhaps because he felt his end to be near: for on the 16th of December,
2 Richard II [1378], the Mayor and Aldermen of London exempted William
atte Vyne "wolmongere" from jury service on account of his great age
(*Calendar* of City Corporation Letter Books *H*, p. 110, edited by R. R.
Sharpe).   [2] See p. 18.

[3] For this identification and further information thereon see Elijah
Williams, *Early Holborn and the Legal Quarter of London* (1927).

[4] *Calendar of Patent Rolls*, 1348–1350, p. 119.

[5] "Heirs", because at this period such land could not be devised by will,
and passed on the death of the tenant thereof to the heir-at-law. (Hence
arose trusts to provide for illegitimate children.) It was otherwise with land

married daughters as co-heirs) and "John de Mirfeld", son of his other sister Margaret.[1]

It is impossible to identify this nephew John as our author, for it is clearly the above-named heir, and not his namesake of the Clerical Subsidy Roll for 1379, who, under the name of "John, son of John de Fournays de Mirfeld", went (on the 25th of October 1351) into the Royal Chancery in London, and acknowledged as his a deed executed at Mirfeld and dated the 24th of October 1351, by which he granted to William de Mirfeld, clerk, all his lands in the "town" of Mirfeld,[2] and who, according to an Inquisitio Post Mortem[3] in which he is described as "John son of John de Fourneys de Mirfeld", died (obviously childless) in 1377, possessed of the manor of Fersley. His heir was his brother Adam, aged upwards of forty years; who, on the 12th of November 1382, obtained a royal licence to transfer the manor of Fersley to Sir Robert de Swyllyngton, Knight (a man who, it may be noted, had business dealings with the surgeon Adam Rous).[4] In this licence Adam de Fourneys de Mirfeld is described as a citizen and goldsmith of London. He lived apparently in the parish of St Peter Westcheap; and he died in 1394 leaving a son named Thomas who was also a London goldsmith and who died in 1407 a few months after John Mirfeld the inhabitant of St Bartholomew's Close.[4]

Although there is no visible link which connects John the possessor of the Mirfeld property in Holborn with Adam, nephew of the priest William de Mirfeld, yet it is obvious that there was at least one branch of William's family resident in London near St Paul's; moreover Thomas Mirfeld alluded

---

situated in London, for this, being held on burgage tenure, was freely devisable. (See R. R. Sharpe, *Calendar of Wills proved and enrolled in the Court of Husting, London*, Part I, 1258–1358, Introduction, p. xxxv (1889).)

[1] See Appendix C, p. 179.   [2] *Calendar of Close Rolls*, 1349–1354, p. 393.
[3] See Appendix C, p. 182.   [4] See Appendix C, pp. 182, 183.

in his will to his kinsmen the brothers Nicholas and Adam
Mirfeld, and Roger de Barnesburgh provided a legacy for
a tailor named Adam de Miryfild[1]; whilst John Mirfeld the
author is sometimes referred to in the Hustings Rolls as
"of Co. York".[2] It seems, therefore, highly probable that
William the Chancery Clerk, and John the author, were
kinsmen, even though possibly remote: for otherwise it is
hardly conceivable that William would have treated John
with such confidence as to make him, in effect, the legatee
of his Holborn property, either as trustee or as the actual
beneficiary, when William's undoubted nephew Adam was
resident close at hand.

The matter can be carried one stage further by turning
again to Bishop Braybroke's Register,[3] where it will be found
that a certain William Mirfeld, of York diocese, was, by
letters dimissory from the authorities of that diocese,
ordained Subdeacon in London on the 23rd of September
1391, on this occasion giving as his title the Hospital of St
Bartholomew, Smithfield; and that when, on the 1st of
March 1393, he was advanced to the priesthood he appears
as incumbent of the parish church of Leeds in Yorkshire.
This living he soon exchanged for that of Swillington, the
patronage of which belonged to the family of the Sir
Robert de Swyllyngton mentioned above.

This second William was also a Chancery clerk, and
almost certainly owed his position to a connection with the
elder William who died in 1375.

Owing to the loss of the Chartulary of the Priory of St
Bartholomew,[4] it is impossible to be certain of what actually
took place: but the foregoing facts suggest that the elder
William de Mirfeld had entered into an arrangement

[1] Appendix C, p. 181.
[2] Roll 107, Nos. 168, 169 (27 May and 1 June, 2 Rich. II [1379]).
[3] See Appendix C, p. 175.
[4] That of the Hospital is happily still in the possession of the Governors.

with the Priory, whereby in return for benefactions which he promised to make in his will, a corrody was to be available for such of his relatives as should apply for it. Although, under the terms of Bishop Sudbury's compromise in 1373, the Priory was no longer responsible for the maintenance of the Hospital, or empowered to superintend the management of its property, it is possible that an agreement was made between the two institutions, whereby the Priory provided a chaplaincy in the Hospital when William Mirfeld the Younger and John the author successively found themselves without the title necessary for ordination to the priesthood.[1]

It has been shown elsewhere[2] that in 1382 John Muryfeld, "clericus", received forty shillings for acting as one of the executors of John Chishull, a chaplain who (as appears from his will) lodged within St Bartholomew's Close and desired to be buried before the altar of St Stephen in the Priory church, to which he was a benefactor. This man is in fact the "Dominus Johannes Chyshull", whose name[3] appears in the Clerical Subsidy Roll of 1379 among the "Clerks of the Priory" of St Bartholomew's, and who paid as his share of the Tax the sum of 2s. It was presumably in the capacity of trustee, in anticipation of this executorship, that Mirfeld appears in company with Chishull as joint donor to the Priory of certain rents in Tewin, Hertfordshire, together with the reversion of Tewin manor, permission to

---

[1] There is one other explanation of the preceding facts, which, however, we advance only tentatively and with reluctance; namely, that the elder William de Mirfeld had, though a Priest, uncanonically married Margaret Schadelok, and was himself the father of John the author. Such marriages, though not unknown among William's colleagues in the Chancery, were officially held invalid, and therefore John would have been incapable of succeeding to William's property. This, too, would account for the rejection of John's first application for ordination if he had neglected to obtain the necessary dispensation. Possibly the corrody was purchased for his maintenance, when he became old enough to enter the Priory of St Bartholomew.

[2] By Webb, *op. cit.* Vol. I, p. 531.

[3] Printed as "Hyshull" by Webb, *op. cit.* Vol. I, p. 172.

acquire the same being given to the Prior by a royal licence dated the 27th of May 1377.[1]

It was perhaps, too, as a trustee that Mirfeld was joined with Robert Brian in making a grant to the Priory (for the maintenance of such charges as John and Robert should order) of three messuages in the parish of St Andrew "in the suburb", two parts of one house and two shops in the parish of St Nicholas Shambles by Ivy Lane together with the reversion of the third part upon the death of Joan, lately wife of Simon atte Gate; and, in addition, the reversion of a house in the parish of St Mary Bow and of another in that of St Sepulchre, Newgate; for the licence to acquire all of which (dated the 28th of June 1392) the Prior had to pay forty pounds to the King.[2] The houses in St Andrew Holborn have been identified as those which Mirfeld obtained from his kinsman William and granted to Herthull, as has been explained above: whilst the other property comprised in the licence, and especially the reversions in the parishes of St Mary Bow and St Sepulchre, which were dependent upon the death of Henry Godechepe, citizen of London (who died in 1394 and was buried in the Priory of St Bartholomew[3]), can be traced back in the Hustings Rolls as purchases of Mirfeld, Brian, Thomas de Maydeston, and the John Chishull mentioned above, evidently on behalf of the last-named person.

Nothing can be found, however, in explanation of the royal licence dated the 20th of September 1392 permitting the acquisition by the Prior from John Mirfeld and John Harpesfeld of the manor of "Walhale" (i.e. Wall Hall in St Stephen's parish) in Hertfordshire, for the maintenance

---

[1] *Calendar of Patent Rolls*, 1374–1377, p. 472; and Webb, *op. cit.* Vol. 1, p. 169.
[2] *Calendar of Patent Rolls*, 1391–1396, p. 102; and Webb, *op. cit.* Vol. 1, p. 182.
[3] His will, dated the 1st of July 1394, was proved in the London Commissary Court. Courtney's Register, f. 328 (Somerset House).

of such charges as the two donors should order.[1] Probably the two men were acting as trustees on behalf of Adam Rous; for the King's Surgeon had bought an annual rent, due on certain property situated in the Parish of All Hallows the Great in the Ropery, from Christina—the widow and executrix of John Harpesfeld, a citizen of London who had died in 1361—to whom he bequeathed a legacy of 6s. 8d. and who was probably the mother of the man associated here with Mirfeld.

It is quite possible, however, that Mirfeld and his colleague in this particular transaction were acting as trustees, not of Adam Rous, but of John Chishull, with whom John Harpesfeld and a certain William Stoteville, Vicar of St Sepulchre's, Newgate, had been associated in a royal licence (dated the 12th of January 1374) for the alienation of certain lands in Acton to the Priory of St Bartholomew, Smithfield.[2] This hypothesis is supported by the fact that John Chishull the Chaplain and John Harpesfeld appear together as partners in the joint ownership of a London brewhouse ("tenementum bracinium") which adjoined certain tenements acquired by John Mirfeld, "Clericus", in company with Thomas de Maydeston and Robert Brian, on the 12th of March, 2 Richard II [1379].[3]

A consideration of the preceding transactions leads to the conclusion that John de Mirfeld was in fact secretly acting as trustee on behalf of William de Mirfeld, Adam Rous and others, and held the property transferred to him for the benefit of St Bartholomew's Priory. The institution of such a trusteeship was the usual method of avoiding the mortmain statutes which forbade gifts of land to religious corpora-

[1] *Calendar of Patent Rolls*, 1391–1396, p. 156; and Webb, *op. cit.* Vol. 1, p. 182. It belonged to the Priory until the Dissolution: the site is now occupied by Aldenham Abbey.
[2] *Calendar of Patent Rolls*, 1370–1374, p. 380.
[3] Hustings Roll 107, no. 116.

tions except by royal licence. Parliament attempted to prevent such evasions of its enactments, and passed a statute in November 1391 (15 Richard II, c. 5) which ordered all persons who held lands in trust for[1] religious and other corporations, either to sell them or else to procure royal licences and convey them in mortmain to the appropriate religious communities before the next ensuing Michaelmas, on pain of forfeiture for non-compliance. It was probably as a result of this statute that Mirfeld showed such activity in obtaining royal licences in mortmain, and conveying land to the Priory of St Bartholomew during the course of the year 1392; a fact which tends to show that Mirfeld was certainly not a member of the monastic body.

Of authenticated evidence concerning John Mirfeld there is little further trace. The date of his birth is uncertain, and for further information pertaining to him, one is forced back upon such vague tradition as that of Leland, who, in his *Commentarii de Scriptoribus Britannicis*, says that "Joannes Marifeldus" lived close by the Hospital of St Bartholomew in London, and that he acquired "immortal fame" for his cures in the London district. Pits has expanded this statement into the assertion that Mirfeld was born in London and lived there all his life.

The assumption that our author was educated at Oxford rests upon no more certain a foundation than a misinterpretation of some notes concerning Mirfeld, which were made by the Oxford antiquary Brian Twyne, and in particular of one passage in the *Breviarium* itself. Twyne borrowed the copy of the *Breviarium Bartholomei* now owned by Pembroke College, Oxford, and made an insertion in the margin of folio 42, at the point where, in describing

---

[1] The modern equivalent of the expression "possessed...to the use of" which occurs in the Statute. Confusion is still often caused by misdating this statute as 1392. Actually the Parliament began on the Morrow after All Souls, 15 Richard II, i.e. November 1391.

jaundice (i.e. Part II, distinction 1, chapter 24, "De Ictericia") Mirfeld mentions a particular remedy and then
continues: "Wherefore Master Nicholas Tyngewich, sitting
in his Chair at Oxford, narrated that he had ridden forty
miles" in order to purchase this specific from a certain
old woman. Brian Twyne's marginal note here, "floruit
hic [Oxford] Tyngewich sub Edw°. 2°", clearly refers to
Tyngewich and not to Mirfeld; nor does Twyne himself
ever claim that Mirfeld was at Oxford; in fact he has inserted the words "Medicus London." above the line immediately following the name of our author in his bio-
graphical collections.[1] It has, however, been inferred from
the passage in the *Breviarium* quoted above (glossed, as it
has been, by a misreading of Twyne's notes) that Mirfeld
was actually present at the lecture when Tyngewich made
his statement. The wording of the passage, however, does
not necessarily imply that our author was himself present
at that moment, and he may possibly have heard the
story from another person, perhaps John Gaddesden the
physician,[2] who certainly was an Oxford man. It is hardly
possible that Mirfeld could have been old enough to have
been himself present, since his mother was still living in
1407; for it is probable that Tyngewich the royal physician
was already dead in the year 1340, when a lease was granted
of the Oxford hall which long bore his name and which he
had purchased in 1302 and had handed over to the University in 1322, retaining for himself, however, a life interest therein.[3] Certainly Tyngewich was no longer living
on the 21st of August 1343 (XII Kalends of September),
for on that day the Pope granted the petition of Henry de

[1] Brian Twyne MS. No. XXII, f. 374 (Oxford University Archives).
[2] Quoted in the Breviarium (see p. 87).
[3] For the details of these transactions, see *Mediaeval Archives of the University
of Oxford*, Vol. I, p. 283 (edited by the Rev. H. E. Salter, M.A., Oxford
Historical Society Publications, Vol. LXX, 1920).

Rosse praying for the benefice of "Colsull" [Coleshill] in the diocese of Salisbury which was void by the death of Tyngewich.[1] Possibly the canard which connects Mirfeld with Oxford originated owing to the confusion of John with the elder William de Mirfeld, Canon of Lincoln, for in the fourteenth century Oxford formed part of the diocese of Lincoln. Possibly indeed it arose from a misconception of the reason for the appearance of a Calendar based on the meridian of Oxford in the Pembroke College copy of the *Breviarium*. The name of Mirfeld does not appear in the University records until about fifty years after the death of our author.

In truth nothing definite has been discovered about Mirfeld's education, either concerning his general literary attainment, or with regard to his specialised interest in Medicine, beyond the fact that we must discard Sir Norman Moore's assertion that he was trained by a skilled London surgeon in favour of the theory that his was possibly a purely academic interest derived solely from books. It would have been reasonable to expect that he had (in accordance with contemporary custom) served an apprenticeship with a medical practitioner, were it not for the fact that he has distinctly stated in his preface to the *Breviarium* that he was not a skilled physician, and, moreover, that he never was a pupil—and this latter statement is one which nobody who has perused some of his pages will venture to dispute. It is true that in the body of his work he sometimes alludes to his "Master": but it can be shown that in more than one such case he is merely quoting from well-known medieval text-books. For example, Sir Norman Moore quoted[2] (from the *Breviarium*, Part IX, distinction 2, chapter

---

[1] See *Calendar of Entries in the Papal Registers relating to Great Britain and Ireland—Petitions to the Pope*, Vol. I, p. 71 (edited by W. H. Bliss, 1896).
[2] *Op. cit.* p. 42.

6, "De Motione Cerebri") as an illustration of Mirfeld's practical training under a skilled London instructor, the treatment followed by "My Master" (for thus Mirfeld describes him) when attending a certain Augustinian Canon, whose head was injured by a fall received whilst endeavouring to mount a horse which reared up and threw its unfortunate rider over the crupper. Sir Norman stated that the Canon in question belonged to St Bartholomew's, Smithfield, although there is nothing in the *Breviarium* to support this assertion. As a matter of fact, the whole of this chapter of Mirfeld's compilation has been copied out verbatim from the corresponding portion of a very famous medieval text-book on Surgery, namely, the *Cirurgia Magna* of Lanfranc of Milan, who died in 1315. In the particular passage quoted (Doctrina III, Tract. II, cap. 1) Lanfranc says that he himself treated this Canon, who resided in the City of Milan; and Mirfeld, when quoting the passage, merely altered Lanfranc's "as I did" into "as my Master did", and left out the important words "of the City of Milan" by which the Canon is described! On no account could Mirfeld have been a pupil of Lanfranc, even when that great surgeon had migrated from Milan to Paris, for the Englishman died nearly a century later than the man whose work he has quoted.

As in the case of Surgery, so too with regard to Medicine, must Mirfeld's references to his "Master" be received with caution, for in the *Breviarium* chapter on Consumption, which will be found printed below, Mirfeld describes a certain test as having been used by his Master. Here again, all that happened was that Mirfeld copied out verbatim a section from the book written by a famous Salernitan physician, Johannes Platearius the Younger (*circ.* 1100), but has changed the "My father" (i.e. J. Platearius the Elder) of Platearius into "My Master". Other instances

of a like kind could doubtless be adduced, were it profitable
to do so: enough has been shown to indicate the nature of
Mirfeld's interest in Medicine, and it is always possible
that his studies in medical literature were initiated and
encouraged by Adam Rous (who would almost certainly
have used Lanfranc's work as one of his text-books), although this did not involve him in any direct practical
instruction.

Conclusion

The aggregate of what has been deposed in the preceding
pages concerning our author seems to warrant the hypo-
theses that, in addition to the facts relating to his life which
we have ascertained and recorded, John de Mirfeld was
indeed a member of the powerful Mirfield family; and that
either he was actually born in London or that he left his
native Yorkshire for the capital, where the support of a relative, who was a courtier, may have procured his connection
with St Bartholomew's, Smithfield. It is probable also that
the same influence secured him an introduction to Adam
Rous, the King's surgeon, who was undoubtedly acquainted with the elder William de Mirfeld whom he must
have met frequently either at the King's court or when in
attendance upon William's patron John of Gaunt; since
it is known from the surgeon's will that the Duke of Lancaster had presented Rous with a girdle, pouch, and knife,
presumably in return for professional services.[1] It may indeed be from Rous that Mirfeld acquired his taste for the
study of Medicine, but it is extremely doubtful, however,
whether he received any regular medical instruction either
from Adam Rous or from anybody else.

The actual nature of Mirfeld's connection with St Bartholomew's is by no means clear. He may perhaps have
acted as an amateur physician in the Priory until his ordina-

---

[1] Bequeathed by Rous to Sir William Stodeleye.

tion, and then have become a chaplain in the Hospital. All that can safely be postulated is that, though not a Canon of the Augustinian Order, he resided within the walls of the Priory: that his conduct as trustee justified the confidence of his friends in his integrity: and that, moved by compassion towards his afflicted fellow-men, he turned to advantage the opportunity afforded him to study in the monastic library, and wrote two books. The first of these, the *Breviarium Bartholomei*, is a purely medical work composed probably between 1380 and 1395, and the second, the *Florarium Bartholomei*, a theological treatise containing one medical chapter, which was probably written at a somewhat later date (see pp. 38 and 102). In these two compilations, named after the House in which he lived, he laboriously gathered together everything that he believed would be conducive to both the physical and spiritual health of mankind, and dedicated it to the service of suffering humanity.

II. JOHANNES DE MIRFELD AS A MEDICAL WRITER

If we turn now from the author himself to a consideration of his works, we find ourselves immediately plunged into that extraordinary welter of ideas, Classical, Arabian, Scholastic, and Magical, the aggregate complexity of which is known as Medieval Medicine. On this subject some general remarks are necessary, if the qualifications and mental environment of the medieval physician are to be made clear to the modern reader.

The peculiar characteristics of the system of Medicine which dominated Western Europe during the Middle Ages were not the results of chance occurrences, but sprang from causes the origins of which were deeply rooted in the pre-

vious history of Europe. Wave after wave of barbarian in-
vasion had shaken the Roman Empire to its foundations,
and those provinces which we are wont to regard as the
home of culture were devastated by successive hordes of
untutored savages. From these and other causes neither
the Eastern nor the Western branch of the Empire was able
to offer a really strong resistance when the followers of
Mohammed swept down upon it, nor could help be expected from the weakened Persian Empire, which was also
over-run. Both Constantinople and Rome were attacked by
the Infidels, and a powerful Moslem empire, which embraced Arabia, Persia, Syria, Egypt, and Spain, was founded
during the eighth century of the Christian era. After
the first flush of conquest was over, the Moslems began to
assimilate the Greek culture of their conquered Byzantine
subjects; not always, however, through the medium of the
original Greek of the authors, but frequently through Syriac
translations of their works. Rendered from the Syriac into
Arabic these works eventually found their way to Western
Christian Europe as translations of the Arabic into Latin,
which remained practically the sole means of access to
them until the Renaissance.

The history of Medicine followed a course similar to that
of the other branches of learning. If the Arabs did not
share the veneration of the Christians for the Golden Age
that was past, they at least agreed with them in their deference to certain great authorities, and thus it was that the
names of Hippocrates of Cos (460 B.C.–*circ.* 377) and his
commentator Galen of Pergamon, "The Prince of
Physicians" (*circ.* A.D. 130–200), dominated Medicine for
more than fifteen hundred years.

Claudius Galen, a physician at the court of the Emperor
Marcus Aurelius, gathered into one vast corpus all the
somewhat discordant elements of Greek medicine, and,

adding thereto his own anatomical knowledge, endeavoured
by means of philosophical reasoning to explain, in terms of
anatomy, the functioning of God in the Universe. It has
been suggested that it was probably this monotheistic
philosophy, rather than his scientific qualifications, which
made Galen acceptable to both Moslem and Christian
alike and ensured the triumph of his medical system. To
so high a degree was the veneration of Hippocrates and
Galen carried that the very words which they wrote (or
were reputed to have written) came to be regarded as
authoritative, and were blindly followed to such an extent
as to distract attention from, and finally to obscure, the
scientific principles which they enshrine. As a result of
this, many medical writers who were doubtful concerning
the success of their forthcoming publications foisted them
upon a gullible world under the name, not of themselves, but
of Hippocrates or Galen. Consequently, an unwieldy mass
of spurious literature parades with such attributions, one
example being the *Capsula Eburnea* quoted by Mirfeld,[1] a
short treatise containing a number of aphorisms, which
received its title from the supposed discovery of the original
manuscript in an ivory box placed inside the tomb of
Hippocrates.

Translated into Arabic by Honain ben Isaac[2] of Baghdad
(*circ.* A.D. 820–873) Galen was soon revered as an authority
by the Arabians, and upon him was based the great work
of Hali Abbas,[3] a Persian who died about A.D. 994, whose
Al-Malikī or *Royal Book* (which recommends attendance at
hospitals to the physician) was translated into Latin by
Constantinus Africanus at Monte Cassino about the year
A.D. 1080, and published by him in a slightly abbreviated
form as his own work under the title of *Pantegni.*

A little previously to Hali Abbas in point of time there

---

[1] See *infra* pp. 62, 63. [2] Ḥunain ibn Isḥāḳ. [3] ʿAlī ibn ʿAbbās.

had lived in Egypt a Jew, Isaac ben Solomon, known as
Isaac Judaeus,[1] who wrote, in Arabic, a book on *Particular Diets*, and whose *Pantegni* is so identical with the
work of Hali Abbas that Hali has been suspected of
foisting Isaac's book upon the world under his own name.

Previous to both in point of time and far superior to them
in learning was the great Rhazes[2] (*circ.* A.D. 868–932), the
"first and foremost of the Arabians" as he has been termed,
who was destined to exercise a profound influence upon the
history of medieval medicine. Of the works attributed to
him one of the most famous was the *Liber Ad Regem Almansorem*: this book was frequently quoted by later authors,
included amongst whom is John Mirfeld.

Following these men comes the Persian Avicenna[3]
(A.D. 980–1037), whose ponderous work, the *Canon*, was
destined to supersede Hali as the text-book of Arabian
medicine. Avicenna, like Galen, partly owed his popularity perhaps to the fact of his being a philosopher, and of
reconciling Galen and Aristotle into one system.

These authors were translated into Latin by either Constantinus Africanus or by Gerard of Cremona, and exercised
a profound influence on medieval medical writing; so that to
quote them blindly became one of the recognised methods
of composing a treatise. These are the chief authorities
who will be met with in those extracts from the works of
Bernardus de Gordonio which figure so prominently in the
compilations of John Mirfeld.

Whilst the Arabians were absorbing and extending the
knowledge of the science of healing, chiefly with regard to
Materia Medica, another focus of medical learning was
beginning to form in the southern Italian town of Salerno,
the medical school of which became so justly famous. Al-

[1] Isḥāḳ ibn Sulaimān.
[2] Abū Bakr Muḥammad ibn Zakarīyā, al-Rāzī.
[3] Husain ibn 'Abd Allāh ibn Sīnā.

though Constantinus Africanus resided near it when he translated his Arabian authors, he is now considered not to have had much influence upon the school, since, although Salerno was under Norman rule when at the height of its greatness, it had previously formed a part of the Byzantine Empire, and its language had been and its traditions were largely Greek, and took as their basis the Hippocratic writings.

Famous for dietetics and hygiene, the school began to rise into prominence about A.D. 1000, and eventually its rules of health became associated together in a Latin poem of some 362 lines, which received the name of the *Schola Salernitana*, or *School of Salerno*, a work which became the most popular medical treatise of the Middle Ages, and which was translated into almost every European vernacular.

The *School of Salerno* was apparently intended for the guidance, not so much of the medical profession, as for that of the general public; a fact which is apparent from the dedication, for the poem opens with the words "Anglorum regi scripsit tota schola Salerni". The "King of the English", who is thus addressed, was formerly considered to be the Crusader, Robert Duke of Normandy, eldest son of William the Conqueror, who, although the rightful King of England according to the law of primogeniture, was never able to secure his inheritance, for he was defeated and captured by his brother King Henry I at the Battle of Tinchebrai, in A.D. 1106, and passed the remainder of his life in captivity. If this identification be admitted, then the poem was written during the visit of Robert to Salerno, in 1099, to be cured of a wound. This traditional ascription is, however, no longer accepted; partly owing to the fact that several manuscripts have been found which begin with the words "Francorum regi", in place of "Anglorum regi", but chiefly on the more impressive ground that modern authorities do not consider the poem to have originated until at least the second half of the thirteenth century.

Concerning the authorship of the *Schola* nothing is known with certainty. It may have been composite, though in medieval days it was ascribed to a certain John of Milan, who was credited with having been the head of the medical faculty at Salerno when the poem was written. Some writers have maintained that the *Schola* was the work of none other than one of its best known commentators, viz. Arnold of Villanova (A.D. 1235–1312), who passed it off as the production of Salerno in order to give it prestige. The poem was considerably expanded during the course of the Middle Ages, but the Villanova version remained the authoritative text, and that which was used by Mirfeld for his quotations in the *Florarium*, although he uses the fuller version in the *Breviarium Bartholomei*.

The literary labours of the members of the medical school of Salerno were not, however, confined to the production of the popular poem which bears its name, for a long and important series of genuinely professional medical works issued from the pens of its disciples (including, for instance, those of Bartholomaeus and the Younger Platearius quoted by Mirfeld). Nor was the influence of the school confined to the district of Salerno itself, for many of the leading exponents of its doctrines lived outside its borders, and quickened medical opinion until Salerno eventually became the recognised centre of the medical learning of Western Europe, and gave its name to the historical period which lasted from the twelfth century until the Renaissance.

Of the many institutions which came into being as a result of the general revival of learning which took place in the twelfth century, the University of Montpellier was destined to become one of the most famous, and of its professors, one, namely Bernardus[1] de Gordonio, to be one of the most widely read of medieval medical text-book writers. Bernardus de Gordonio became professor in the year A.D. 1285 and he produced a number of well known works, the most famous of which is his *Lilium Medicine*, completed in 1305, which long held place as one of the best modern books of its day, and continued to be printed until the seventeenth century. It is this famous exemplar of medieval medicine which Mirfeld quotes so copiously in the medical, as distinct from the surgical, section of the *Breviarium*; so that a study of Bernardus forms the best introduction which can be given to the theories of our author.

Bernardus was an original thinker and experimenter, but his mental horizon was too closely bounded by the Scholastic philosophy of his day, based upon the newly discovered Aristotle; consequently, when expounding his medical doctrines, he could not escape from the medieval practice of quoting authorities. His custom, indeed, was first to marshal an array of conflicting and authoritative opinions, and then, only after explaining them away, did he venture to assert his own. His advice was naturally founded upon the peculiar physiological and pathological theories of his day which had descended to him from Galen by way of the Arabians; and this "humoral pathology", as it is termed, demands some explanation.

According to medieval ideas the body was endowed with "natural" or innate heat, situated in the liver, which digested the food contained in the stomach, the process being likened to the cooking of food in a cauldron over the fire. In the first stage of the digestive process, the food underwent a series of successive refinements in the stomach and intestines, the purer part, in each case, being chiefly carried

[1] He is the physician "Bernard" mentioned in Chaucer's "Prologue".

as "chyle" to the hilum of the liver;[1] and there what was known as the "second digestion" took place, in which the four "humours" or fluids were generated in substance and then sent to the appropriate organs to receive their special forms.

These four humours were: firstly, the blood, which was formed in the liver; secondly, the phlegm, which came from the lungs, brain, and stomach; thirdly, the yellow bile, formed in the gall bladder; and lastly, the black bile, which was generated in the spleen. (In the final, or "third digestion", the blood in the liver was carried from it by the veins to the various parts of the body, and then transformed into flesh, skin and bone.)

The four humours thus generated were considered to enter into combination with those fundamental qualities of heat, cold, moisture and dryness, which were the attributes of the "Four Elements" of fire, air, water, and earth; and that, too, in such a manner, that blood was considered to be hot and moist, phlegm cold and moist, yellow bile hot and dry, and black bile cold and dry. It was a superfluity of one of these humours in the body of a man that was held to be the origin of disease, for health could exist only if there were an even balance of the humours, or "temperament",[2] as it was termed. An excess of one humour would, according to this theory, obviously be accompanied by a corresponding shortage of the others; and the proportion in which this existed in the body was termed its "complexion", of which four well-defined types were recognised, each one of which corresponded to a superfluity of one of the humours. Thus a man possessed of excess of "blood" was said to be "sanguine" in complexion, one troubled with

---

[1] Some was retained for nourishment.
[2] "Non est sanitas nisi per equalitatem complexionum et non est equalitas complexionis nisi per temperanciam humorum" (*Secretum Secretorum*).

too much phlegm was called "phlegmatic"; whilst an excess of yellow bile gave rise to the "choleric", and of black bile to the "melancholic" of complexion.

Not only was each of these four humours held to be the predisposing cause of certain types of physical disease, but they were also considered to have some connection with the emotions, the effects of which on the body were also noticed; and to such an extent was this theory carried that the mental outlook, and indeed, the psychical functioning, of a man were considered to depend upon the particular humour prevalent in him, until the term "complexion" became part of the vocabulary of the non-medical public and synonymous with "characteristic".

Since the possession of health depended in theory upon the maintenance of the balance of the humours in the body, disease was treated by supplying the patient with food and medicine containing matter of an opposite nature to that of his prevailing humour. For this purpose an elaborate scheme was evolved by means of which the various qualities inherent, according to the "humoral" theories, in various forms of food, drink, and medicine, were noted down and tabulated for ready reference. Account, too, had to be taken of the effects of climate, and of various types of occupation; and added to all of the aforesaid was the idea that those who possessed more "natural heat" (which varied with age, etc.) could digest more easily than those who were not so fortunate. Therefore the medieval physician had perforce to work out an elaborate system of permutations and combinations, in order that, by means of diet and medicines, he might provide his patients with those qualities which were needful to their complexions. The lines along which he worked, and the probability or otherwise of his success, can be gauged by the extracts from Mirfeld's works which we now submit.

Here, then, in these pages will be found recorded the medical knowledge laboriously acquired by a man who, in the days of Richard II, lived in the medieval Priory and was connected with the Hospital of St Bartholomew in Smithfield, and who was acquainted, perhaps intimately, with the King's surgeon, Adam Rous. Elementary and even childish as much of what is contained here will seem to us now in the light of our modern knowledge, and demonstrably futile when confronted, for example, with so, terrible a pestilence as the Black Death, it must nevertheless be remembered that such were the genuine medical doctrines accepted and enshrined in their works by leading writers of the day, and upon which, as the best available, practice in St Bartholomew's and similar Hospitals was based some five hundred years ago. As such these extracts from John de Mirfeld's writings seem worthy of being placed on record, presenting as they do a comparison between the standard of scientific knowledge attained in the Middle Ages with that enjoyed in more modern times, since physicians have learnt from Harvey "to search out and study the secrets of Nature by way of experiment", and from Sydenham the Art of Clinical Medicine.

§ II
The Breviarium Bartholomei

II

THE *BREVIARIUM BARTHOLOMEI*

I. INTRODUCTORY REMARKS

THE FIRST OF MIRFELD'S WORKS with which we propose to deal is the great medical compilation known as the *Breviarium Bartholomei* upon which rests his claim to be regarded as a physician. This book is in form a great encyclopaedia of genuine contemporary medical knowledge, to which has been added much superstitious and magical lore, such as charms and incantations. It is written in Latin, but does not pretend to learning or originality: in fact, its author disclaims the name of physician, and merely desires to be considered as a man who had, from charitable motives, compiled a prescription-book for the use of those whose poverty prevented them from acquiring medical knowledge by one of the usual medieval methods of obtaining it, namely the provision of a suitable library. It is upon this basis that the book is compiled: it contains almost no anatomy, very little of the theory so beloved by medieval writers on Medicine, and only just sufficient indication of the various symptoms (as then understood) to enable a rough and ready diagnosis to be made by a practitioner ignorant of auscultation and percussion, and unacquainted with a thermometer. The whole interest of the compiler centres itself around his proffered remedies, of which a list is provided for each disease, without any enquiry as to whether the prescriptions recommended be good, bad, or indifferent, or any indication as to the schools of thought from which they originate or the theories underlying their use.

The complete text of the work, consisting of Prologue, Epilogue, and Parts I–XV, has survived only in two manuscript copies, both of which were perhaps written during Mirfeld's lifetime. One of these is Harley MS. No. 3 in the British Museum; whilst the other, which is the finer copy, is that owned by Pembroke College, Oxford (MS. No. 2). This latter manuscript contains, at the end of the text above mentioned, the only copy of the *Sinonoma Bartholomei* in existence, and which has been edited, as has already been explained, by Mowat. Immediately following the *Sinonoma* (at f. 348 b) is a section entitled "Quid pro Quo", which provides a list of various drugs and medicines to be used in place of others which may not be available. It is probably based upon the corresponding section of the *Antidotary* of Nicolaus Salernitanus (12th cent. A.D.). At the end of the "Quid pro Quo" will be found the little note on the weights of drugs which is now printed; and which, together with the "Quid pro Quo", appears only in the Pembroke College manuscript.

Moreover, to the text of the *Breviarium Bartholomei* contained in the Pembroke College manuscript is prefixed an astronomical calendar, extracts from which were printed by Mowat with his edition of the *Sinonoma*. Mowat thought this Calendar to be the perpetual calendar made by Walter de Elvesden, and its date to be the year 1387. Sir Norman Moore therefore assumed that the Calendar in the Pembroke College manuscript was made in the year 1387, and that the *Breviarium Bartholomei* must necessarily have been written previous to this date.

It is clear, however, that this theory cannot be upheld. It is evident that Mowat was misled into describing the Calendar as the work of Elvesden owing to the inclusion of the "Canon" (or introduction) to Elvesden's perpetual calendar among the explanatory remarks with which it is prefaced. Nor was the Calendar actually made in the year 1387: for although the Introduction states that it was composed in the year of the Lord "millesimo ccc^{mo} octogesimo septimo", in fact the word "septimo" was added later, thus proving that the date as originally written was 1380, which is the generally accepted date of the calendar ascribed to John Somer.

From an inspection of the Pembroke College manuscript, we have no hesitation in asserting that the astronomical calendar contained in it is none other than that based on the meridian of Oxford and composed in 1380 by the Franciscan John Somer (or Somour), for Joan, Princess of Wales, the mother of Richard II. It consists of a calendar which takes as its basis the year 1387 (in which the date of Easter was the 7th of April and the Dominical letter was F) and contains tables of conjunctions, together with eclipses of the sun and moon, for the period 1387–1462.

So extensively used was Somer's calendar, that its inclusion in the Pembroke College manuscript of the *Breviarium Bartholomei* offers no proof that it was ever intended to form part of Mirfeld's book: and if the occurrence of the medical and astronomical works in the same manuscript is to possess any significance whatsoever, it cannot imply more than that the *Breviarium* was not finished until after the conclusion of Somer's labours. In fact, in this respect, the manuscript offers very little assistance in forming a conclusion.

As, however, it is our bounden duty to supply a date for the composition of the *Breviarium Bartholomei*, it seems reasonable, in default of more definite information, to suggest that the work was composed at a date subsequent to the completion of Somer's calendar, but previous to the ordination of John Mirfeld as a priest, and that it was thus, in fact, written at some time between the years 1380 and 1395.

In his report on the Pembroke College MSS.,[1] H. T. Riley pointed out the authorship of the work from the rubric with which the text of the *Breviarium* in the Pembroke College manuscript opens, viz. (at folio 11):

Incipit liber qui intitulatur Breuiarium Bartholomei compositus per venerabilem virum Johannem Mirfeld commorantem in Monasterio Sancti Bartholomei Londonie a quo liber iste denominatur.

Here beginneth the book called the "Breviary of Bartholomew", which was compiled by the venerable man John Mirfeld, a sojourner within the monastery of St Bartholomew in London, from whence the title of the book is derived.

Riley also noted the fact that on folio 353 appears another rubric, which introduces the table of chapters, viz.:

Incipit tabula libri Johannis Mirfeld quem ipse composuit et breuiarium Bartholomei nominauit eo quod ipsum compilauit in monasterio sancti Bartholomei Londonie, eundemque diuisit in partes quindecim.

Here beginneth the Table of contents to the book of John Mirfeld, which he composed and called the "Breviary of Bartholomew" because he wrote it in the Monastery of St Bartholomew in London; and he divided it into fifteen parts.

Neither of these rubrics occurs in Harley MS. No. 3; but Sir Norman Moore, in his Fitz-Patrick lecture, pointed out that the Harleian manuscript contains, as a footnote on folio 21 b, the following Latin couplet, which Sir Norman could not find in the Oxford copy (but which actually occurs therein on f. 25 b, inserted in the body of the text at the end of the chapter-list preceding Part II and before the opening chapter thereof[2]), and which had hitherto been overlooked:

Ordine pretacto si connumeres capitales
Nomen factoris demonstrabunt tibi tales.

[1] Royal Commission on Historical Manuscripts, Report VI, Part I (1877), Appendix, p. 550.
[2] Actually the opening phrase of Part II, viz.: "Ordinem pretactum vt obseruemus post completam primam partem, etc." immediately precedes the list of chapters. In the Pembroke College MS. then comes the couplet, after which follows the chapter "De Lepra", the first letter (R) of the opening word of which ("Rogerus") provides the second letter of the acrostic, viz. O R (A).

This, being interpreted, enjoins the reader to copy out the first letter of each chapter from this point onwards (i.e. from the beginning of Part II, of which "Ordinem pretactum" form the opening words), whereupon the name of the author will appear. Sir Norman showed that the resulting sentence is as follows:

Ora pro nobis sancte Bartholomee ait Iohannes dde Mirfeld vt digni efficiamur promissionibus Cristi.

"Pray for us, O Holy Bartholomew, says John de Mirfeld, that we may be made worthy of the promises of Christ."

Sir Norman also pointed out that a similar acrostic runs through the *Florarium*, thus linking together the authorship of the two works.[1]

It is a pity, however, that Sir Norman, having ventured thus far, should have believed that he had arrived at the end of the *Breviarium* acrostic, and should have refrained from copying out the initial letters of the chapters following the word "Cristi": for although in the *Florarium* the end of the acrostic coincides with that of the book itself, this is not the case with the *Breviarium*, where the acrostic continues to a great length, and consists of the following invocation and prayer (which will be found written out in full on f. 302 b of Harley MS. No. 3). A modification of this prayer, for use by a patient when taking medicine, was quite common in Mirfeld's day:

Ora pro nobis sancte Bartholomee ait Iohannes dde Mirfeld[2] vt digni efficiamur promissionibus Cristi.

    Oremus.

Deus qui mirabiliter creasti hominem et mirabilius redemisti Et dedisti medicinam ad reparandam sanitatem humanorum corporum: Da omnibus secundum tenorem huius voluminis fideliter operantibus prosperitatem et effectum bonum ad[3] laudem nominis tuui dominee vt famuli

---

[1] See *infra* p. 100.

[2] "S" for "d" in Pembroke College MS. owing to "sicit" being mistakenly written for "dicit" as the first word of Part III, Dist. 1, Cap. 10.

[3] "S" for "d" in Pembroke College MS. "Sicunt" written for "dicunt" as the first word of Part VI, Dist. 1, Cap. 7.

tui quacumque infirmitate vexati[1] per modum medendi hic anotatum conualescant et perfectam sanitatem recipiant vt graciarum tibi referant acciones per cristum dominum nostrum. Amen. Explicit.

which is, being interpreted:

"Pray for us, O Holy Bartholomew, says John de Mirfeld, that we may be made worthy of the promises of Christ.

Let us pray!

O God who hast marvellously created man and more marvellously hast redeemed him, and hast given Medicine to restore the health of human bodies: Grant to all who practise faithfully according to the tenor of this volume a prosperous proceeding and a happy result: so that Thy Name may be praised, O Lord, and that Thy servants, by whatever disease they may be troubled, may, by the manner of healing here set forth, attain to recovery and receive again their perfect health, and render thanks to Thee: through Christ our Lord. Amen. The end."

Incidentally, an excellent idea of the immense size of the *Breviarium* can be gathered from the fact that each letter of the preceding Latin prayer represents one chapter of the book, and that the portion of the compilation thus covered by the acrostic extends only from the beginning of Part II as far as Part IX, distinction 7, chapter 4, of a book which is divided into fifteen parts.[2]

It was not to be expected that John de Mirfeld, when he sat down to compile a prescription-book for those who were not medical experts, should endeavour to produce an original treatise. Indeed, he disclaims all intention of so doing[3]; for, apart from the labour involved, he would thus have vitiated all hope of investing his work with any authoritative attributes, and he therefore confines himself to copying wholesale from the standard medical books of his day.

To produce the full list of his sources would involve writing a bibliography of practically the whole of medieval medical literature, and we must content ourselves, there-

[1] "Vexaci" for "vexati" in Pembroke College MS. "Cenetur" written for "tenetur" as the first word of Part VII, Dist. 3, Cap. 2.

[2] We may add that in Harley MS. No. 3 the chapter "De Ptisi" represents only one three-hundredth part of the volume.

[3] See p. 95.

fore, with indicating here and later those books upon which
are based the extracts from his works now printed.

In the unwieldy mass of Greek medical literature, extant
in Rome during the first century of the Christian era, the
corpus of writings, ascribed to Hippocrates of Cos, occupied a deservedly important place, and claimed the re-
spectful allegiance of Galen, their commentator. Upon
these authorities the Arabians based their works, and
although they originated many new prescriptions, yet they
seem to have never entirely abandoned the notion that
they were but humble disciples following in the footsteps of
great masters, whom they were bound to revere, imitate,
and quote, but never attempt to overthrow.

The fashion thus set naturally appealed to the medieval
physicians, into whose hands the Latin translations of the
Arabians fell, hidebound as they were by precedent and
deference to established authority. It is obvious that books
on so technical a subject as Medicine must, during a given
period, follow upon generally similar lines: but this does
not necessarily involve the plagiarism of the medieval text-
books, in the production of which one of the recognised
methods employed came to consist merely in the arrangement of excerpts from authors of reputation, copied out
blindly, and without any attempt at verification, and
strung together according to medieval notions of logical
arrangement. It is on lines such as these that John de
Mirfeld composed his works.

The construction of the *Breviarium* is that common to many
medieval medical books. It commences with an introduction (of which we shall give a translation), in which Mirfeld
sets forth the reasons which led him to compose the treatise.
Then come sections devoted to illnesses of a general nature,
such as fevers, etc., and after this the diseases are dealt with
according to that part of the body which they affect, commencing with the head, and proceeding downwards to the

feet. The work is divided into fifteen parts, and each part into several "distinctions", and these again into chapters.

The treatise on "The Signs of Death" which is here printed forms one of the chapters (19) of that part of the *Breviarium* dealing with fevers (viz.Part I, distinction 6). It exists also in a separate treatise containing additional matter, but in a hopelessly corrupt form, as Lambeth Palace Library MS. No. 444, f. 180. It is of interest since it provides an example on a small scale of the curious mixture of science, nonsense, and superstition which is presented by Medieval Medicine. It opens with an extract from the *Prognostics* of Hippocrates, including the well-known description of the "Hippocratic Face", and then quotes that part of the *School of Salerno* relating to the signs of death: it returns again to Hippocrates, and then proceeds with excerpts from Book x of Rhazes' *Liber Ad Regem Almansorem*, Avicenna's *Canon*, and other standard works. In the final section, which is not found in either of the two complete MSS. of the *Breviarium* but only in the Lambeth manuscript, the text plunges into a mass of unsavoury nonsense and superstitious magic which was probably inherited from Pagan sources. An inaccurate version of the so-called *Secrets of Hippocrates* then follows, and the treatise ends with a quotation from the *School of Salerno*.

The chapter on "Consumption" is taken from that section which is concerned with diseases of the chest (viz. Part IV, dist. 1), and exemplifies the knowledge and methods of our author when dealing with a particular disease. It opens with a verbatim extract from the *Practica* of a well-known writer, Bartholomaeus of Salerno. It then quotes another Salernitan writer, the younger Johannes Platearius, with the important difference that Mirfeld substitutes "My Master" for "My Father", as the originator of one of the tests for consumption. The rest of the chapter consists chiefly of haphazard extracts from Bernard Gordon's *Lilium Medicine* (a book which incorporates Hippocrates,

Galen, Avicenna, and others) arranged without regard to
their correct order or the explanations necessary to make
them comprehensible, and without any mention of the
"hill treatment" of Galen which is quoted by Gordon.
Possibly Mirfeld had never seen a mountain, or considered
it impracticable to send a London patient to one, and
therefore ignored the matter.

In addition to copious extracts from writers of repute,
the book contains a number of prescriptions and suggestions which are based probably on Pagan magic, and
some of which would be unprintable. Many of these are
actually taken from books bearing the names of well-known
medieval authors where they are frequently found, a large
number of charms and incantations being based on the
writings of Gilbertus Anglicus. The wording of some of the
charms consists of Christian prayers, and Sir Norman
Moore has suggested that the repetition of such a charm or
prayer whilst preparing medicine was in fact a method of
reckoning the time required for each operation. Whatever
their origin, these charms hold a definite place in medieval
medicine, and our author copied them all into his book.
Occasionally, however, he appears to have had some
qualms as to their efficacy in spite of medieval credulity;
for there is one passage in the *Breviarium*, at the end of
chapter 11 of Part VI, distinction 3 ("De difficultate
partus"), where he gives the wording of a prayer, which is
to be written out and tied upon the pregnant woman to
assist delivery of the child, and then adds that, although
some men have faith in such things, he himself holds them
in scant estimation ("Quidam fiduciam habent in talibus,
et forte illis valebunt. Sed non multum sapiunt in iecore
meo, parcat michi deus!"). It may possibly have been this
remark, coupled with his recipes for contraceptives (which,
however, are given in cypher), that led to his rejection the
first time he applied for ordination.

The choice of the extracts from the *Breviarium* which are now printed was necessarily of an arbitrary nature, and was governed by the following considerations. The Prologue and Epilogue contain a general discussion of the nature of the work, and of the reasons for its publication, and provide clues to the personality of the author. For these reasons it has been decided (as in the case of the *Florarium*) to print them in full.

The chapter on the Signs of Death is adduced because it is probably the most general of the sections of the work, and deals with an aspect which is common to many diseases treated, viz. death: moreover, the connection between the Lambeth Palace MS. No. 444 (which Tanner regarded as a separate work) and the *Breviarium* can thus be shown, and this manuscript brought within the orbit of the present publication.

When it was decided to offer one particular disease as an exemplification of Mirfeld's treatment, the choice of the editors was naturally directed to the chapter on "Consumption", partly because of the importance of the subject itself, partly because of their personal interest in all matters relating to this disease, and, lastly, because this particular malady is believed to have caused the death of Mirfeld's great contemporary, the Black Prince, and it was thought that an exposition of the treatment very probably accorded to that famous man would not be without interest in these modern days.

The other items printed are on matters of more general interest. The extract on "Weights and Measures" shows the early use of the apothecaries' two measures: whilst the prescription for making Gunpowder, although perhaps somewhat out of place in a work devoted to the Healing Art, is included on account of its antiquity.

The recipe entitled "Emplastrum Bartholomei" we print for reasons of sentiment.

II. *PROEMIUM*

BREVIARIUM BARTHOLOMEI

In principio huius compilacionis sicut in omnibus operibus
nostris deo gratias agamus sicut sui status celsitudo et bene-
ficiorum ipsius exigit multitudo. De cuius bonitate con-
fidens quasdam notabilitates medicinales quas in diuersis
locis textuum et glossarum artis medicine necnon et in
opusculis plurimorum de ista sciencia subtiliter et copiose
tractancium inueni et collegi quas nunc tenet labilis memoria mea hortatu quorundam amicorum meorum iuxta
ingenii mei modulum sub quodam compendio collocare
disposui; ne, si semel a predicta mea breui memoria pro-
labantur, non possent de facili iterum a tam rudi collectore
reuocari vt possint semel collecte tamquam in modico
seruatorio faciliter reperiri. Sed quoniam istud negocium
non est leue mihi quem multa peccata prepediunt et
euidens ignorancia deprimit domini dei mei gratiam et
auxilium inuoco qui est bonorum omnium principium et
finis Ipsumque idem obsecro vt huic mee compilacioni
principium bonum et finem congruum concedat. Meque
custodiat ne quid in ea scribatur vel dicatur quod voluntati
sue displiceat vel quod alicui suorum cedat ad nocumentum.

Sed forsitan aliquis mihi dicet Quomodo te preparas ad
scribendum quid non debite didicisti, nec agnouisti adhuc
formam discipuli? Vnde non videris attendere quid commentator super Viaticum dicit. Sola, inquit, medendi est
ars quam sibi omnes passim vendicant hanc vniuersi pre-
sumunt lacerant atque docent. Consideres ergo quid dicit
beatus Jeronimus scribens ad Rusticum Monachum. Ad

THE PREFACE

BREVIARIUM BARTHOLOMEI

In the beginning of this compilation, as in all our labours, let us
offer to God the thanks due to His excellent greatness and to the
multitude of His mercies; in whose goodness confiding, I have
found and gathered together certain noteworthy matters of a
medical nature culled from various sources, such as texts and
glosses of the Art of Medicine, as well as the works of many writers
who have treated of this science skilfully and fully; and, since
I now merely retain these things in my mind, from whence they
are prone to slip away, I have endeavoured, at the instigation
of certain of my friends, and according to my ability, to collect
them together and to set them down in an abridged form;
partly because if once they are allowed to slide away from my
aforesaid short memory they cannot easily be recovered again
by so unskilled a student as myself, and partly because when
once brought together, as it were, into a storehouse of moderate
size, they may easily be found.

Since, however, this task is not a light one to me (for the
multitude of my errors embarrasses me, and my evident ignorance weighs me down) I earnestly implore the grace and help
of the Lord my God, who is the beginning and the end of all
goodness; and I pray that He will grant me a good beginning
and a worthy ending to this my compilation, and that He will
preserve me from writing or saying anything which will be dis-
pleasing to Him, or which will be productive of harm to any
of His people.

Peradventure, however, somebody will say to me, "How can
you make ready to write about a subject in which you have
never received proper instruction, and have not known hitherto
what it means to occupy the position of a pupil? From this
you would appear to heed not the words of the Commentator
on the 'Viaticum'[1] when he says, 'The Art of Healing is the
only one which all men everywhere appropriate to themselves,
and which they all pretend to know, mangle, and expound!'
You should consider, therefore, what the blessed Jerome says,
when, writing to the monk named Rusticus, he thus addresses
him:

[1] "Incipit liber viatici a Constantino Cassiniensis". According to Mr Fulton
of the British Museum, the Viaticum peregrinantis of Constantinus Africanus is really only his translation from the Arabic of the *Zād al-Musāfir* or
"Traveller's provisions" by Ibn al-Jazzār. The "commentator" is Gerard
of Cremona (*c.* A.D. 1150).

scribendum,inquit, cito non prosilias et leui ducaris insania, sed multo tempore disce quid doceas.

Ad istam quidem obieccionem breuiter et veraciter possum respondere meum recognoscendo defectum. Quoniam non decet me scribere tamquam docturum sed si velim ad labilitatem mee memorie supportandam quasdam notabilitates medicinales collectas in vno breuiario conscribere quod tanquam promptuarium mihi fiat non credo quod debeat aliquis rationabiliter inde mihi inuidere. Sed si rudis sit lector sicut et ego mecum si velit participet de collectis, sin autem in ista scientia sit precellens qui rudem hanc collectam respexerit parcat obliuioso sibi prouidere volenti Et euellat si velit inconueniencia et addat meliora. Quidem enim tanti operis vtilitatem temptaui tractare et ordine certo doctorum precedencium sententias sub compendio redigere desideraui, plus fuit ex desiderio simplicioribus mihi similibus proficiendi quam ex cupiditate alicuius inanis iactancie procurande Que circa prouidus lector simplicitati compilatoris parcat corrigendo Et discat potius deliberata ratione emendare quam inuidie liuore dilacerando detrahere.

Alia etiam subest causa scribendi presencia. Frequenter enim mihi accidit vt aut propter meam aut propter amicorum meorum infirmitatem varias fraudes modernorum medicorum experirer. Quidam enim illorum ea que curare nesciebant cupiditatis causa curare se promittebant. Quidam etiam pro medicinis modice valoris et efficacie multa impudenter exigebant. Nonnullos etiam comperi qui languores quos paucissimis diebus possent repellere in longum tempus protraxerunt vt pacientes diu sibi tributarios haberent Quare propter necessitatem mihi videbatur et vtile vt vndique valetudinis remedia collecta velut in vno

'Do not speedily blossom forth as an author, or be led away by your light-minded enthusiasm; but receive instruction for a long time, so that you may be able to teach what is correct'"!"

I can, indeed, briefly and truthfully reply to this objection, by admitting my own shortcomings; for it is not fitting that I should write in the manner of one about to teach: but if, in order to provide a support for my unreliable memory, I should desire to gather together certain noteworthy medical facts and to write them all together into one breviary so that this may serve as a repository for me, I do not believe that anybody ought reasonably to look askance at me upon such an account. If, however, the reader be as ignorant as I am, he may, if he so wishes, participate with me in the enjoyment of this collection. If, on the contrary, there shall gaze upon my clumsy compilation an individual, who is highly distinguished in this branch of knowledge, let him be merciful to one who, because of his own liability to forget, desires to take precautions for himself; and let him, if he will do so, erase what is unsuitable, and add something better.

I have essayed to give utility to the work by arranging it in a methodical manner. My object, in wishing to reduce the opinions of the most distinguished teachers into one abridgement, was more the desire of assisting simpletons such as myself, than any passion to indulge in empty-headed ostentation. Wherefore, let the prudent reader spare the simpleness of the compiler by correcting the book and let him learn to amend its faults with mature deliberation, rather than to detract from its merits by hatefully and spitefully tearing it to pieces.

There is also another reason for writing this book.[2] It has frequently happened that I have experienced the fraudulent practices of modern physicians, either when I myself needed their services, or when my friends were ill. Some of these practitioners were led by avarice to promise that they would cure a disease concerning which they were ignorant. Some impudently exacted a high price for medicines of little efficacy or intrinsic value: whilst others of the breed protracted the treatment over a considerable period, in cases where the infirmity could have been healed within a few days, just in order that they might have their patients as tributaries for a long time. Wherefore it seemed to me that it was both necessary as well

---

[1] Printed among the works of St Jerome as Epistle No. cxxv in Migne, *Patrologia Latina*, xxii, 1072.

[2] The opening section of this paragraph seems based on the "Epistula Plinii Secundi ad amicos de Medicina" incorporated amongst the "Epistulae diversorum de qualitate et observatione Medicinae" forming the introduction to the *De Medicamentis* of Marcellus Empiricus (fifth century A.D.).

breuiario vt predictum est conscriberem Vt quocunque
venirem huiusmodi impostores vitare possem et vt mihimet
ipsi et Christi pauperibus scirem mederi si in languoribus
curabilibus et lenibus incidere oporteret. Hoc tamen con-
siderare non omittas quoniam medicine actio secundum
proprietatem subiecti frequenter immutatur; propterea
multas medicinas pro vna et eadem infirmitate ponere
propono in multis locis istius compilacionis. Quoniam de
proprietate medicaminum est quod iuuabunt vno tempore et non alio. Et hoc est mirabile. Et forte facit hoc
varietas proprietatis adquisite ex influencia orbis alicuius.
Preterea scire te volo quod in multis locis opusculi huius
experimentis vti propono, tum quia breuiter expediunt
tum quia multi infirmi modernis temporibus valde im-
pacientes sunt Nolunt enim sicut antiquitus facere solebant
expectare vsque ad quartum vel quintum diem vel amplius
si necesse fuerit, quousque materia peccans fuerit digesta
et vtiliter euacuata. Verum nisi statim in prima die sentiant
alleuiamen de medico diffidunt eiusque medicinas respuunt
et contempnunt. Et intellige quod duplex est experimentum
scilicet experimentum vallatum ratione et experimentum
non vallatum ratione. De primo dicitur quod experimentum est illud quod a prudentibus ratione est inuentum et
huius hic vti intendimus. Experimentum autem si non
sit vallatum ratione tunc timorosum est et fallax vt dicit
Ypocras et Johannes Damascenus.

Verum quoniam in qualibet arte diffusio fastidium
generat ingenii acumen hebetat et memoriam perturbat.
Insuper et res quelibet per diuisionem partium magis
patet. Et vt dicit philosophus in libro de memoria magis
sunt reminiscibilia quecumque ordinacionem aliquam

---

¹ I.e. the unorthodox or untried remedies. (Avicenna, Canon II, i, cap. 2.)
² This refers to the opening words of the *Aphorisms*. Mirfeld being un-
acquainted with the Greek text relied upon the medieval Latin version or
Antiqua Translatio, by Constantinus Africanus, of the Arabic version of

as useful that I should (as has been said above) write down within one breviary the various remedies applicable to each disease; so that, wherever I might come, I might by this means be able to escape impostors of this kind, and might be able to relieve, not only myself, but all the other poor followers of Christ, who should happen to be afflicted by those diseases which are not serious but curable. Nor should one omit here the consideration of how the action of a medicine is frequently changed according to the peculiar nature of the subject for treatment: therefore I propose, in a good many cases, to set down in this compilation several medicines for one and the same disease, since it is a peculiarity of medicaments that at one time they are beneficial, and at another time they are not—a fact which is a matter for wonder! This diversity of effect is perhaps due to the influence of a man's natal planet.

Moreover, I wish it to be known, that in many instances in this compilation, I propose to make use of experiments[1], both because they are speedy in operation, and because many patients in these modern days are particularly impatient, and are unwilling to wait until the fourth or fifth day or more for the morbid matter in the body to be digested and usefully evacuated, as was the custom in the olden days: for in truth, unless such people feel relief immediately on the first day, they distrust their physician and despise and reject his prescriptions.

And note that the significance of the word "experiment" is twofold, namely, an experiment deriving its strength from reason, or one which lacks this quality. Of the former it is said that an experiment is that which has been discovered by the intelligence of prudent men, and it is with this type alone that we propose to deal here: but an experiment, which has not been thus approved, is fearsome and deceptive, as both Hippocrates[2] and John Damascene[3] maintain.

Since, indeed, in any kind of treatise, prolixity begets aversion, dulls the acuteness of the intellect, and confuses the memory; and since, moreover, the nature of anything becomes more obvious by its divisions into sections; and, as the Philosopher[4] says in his book on "The Memory", those things, which possess an ordered arrangement, are easiest recalled to mind:

Ḥunain ibn Isḥāḳ, which begins "Vita Breuis, Ars vero longa Tempus autem acutum experimentum fallax", and misunderstood the words "experimentum fallax".

[3] I.e. Johannes filius Mesue (Yūḥannā ibn Māsawaih, A.D. 777–857). The reference is probably to the Latin translation of his Aphorisms ".... Rerum proprietas dubia est. Ecce namque multi olim experientes arbitrati sunt facere".

[4] I.e. Aristotle.

habent, idcirco presentem compilacionem quam Breuiarium Bartholomei vocari cupio in quindecim partes prin-
cipales dignum duxi diuidendam.

Et ponam vnicuique parti propria capitula Vt quid
inquiritur facilius possit inueniri.

Quare in parte prima auxiliante gratia Christi tracta-
bitur de febribus. In secunda de morbis aliis vniuer-
salibus occupantibus totum corpus vel saltem maiorem
partem corporis. Pars tertia erit de infirmitatibus totius
capitis colli et gule vsque ad superiorem partem pectoris.
Pars quarta erit de infirmitatibus totius clibani pectoris et
contentorum ibidem et etiam brachiorum et manuum.
Pars quinta erit de infirmitatibus corporis a pectore vsque
ad membra genitalia. Pars sexta erit de infirmitatibus
membrorum genitalium. Pars septima erit de infirmitatibus ab ano vsque ad extremam partem pedis vtriusque.
Pars octaua erit de apostematibus. Pars nona erit de
vulneribus cum suis pertinentiis. Pars decima de fractura
ossium. Pars vndecima de dislocatione iuncturarum. Pars
duodecima de medicinis simplicibus. Pars tertia decima
de medicinis compositis. Pars quarta decima de laxatiuis et
purgationibus humorum nociuorum. Pars quinta decima
de fleobotomia et regimine sanitatis et de multis aliis vt
inferius patebit.

therefore, I have considered it advisable to divide this present
compilation (which I desire should be known as the *Breviary
of Bartholomew*) into fifteen principal parts, and to subdivide
each of these into appropriate chapters, so that whatever is
sought may the more readily be found.

Wherefore, in the first part, I shall, with the grace of Christ
helping me, treat of fevers: in the second, of all the other general
diseases which attack the whole body, or at least, the greater
portion of the body. The third part will deal with the infirmities
of the whole of the head, neck, and throat, as far down as the
upper part of the chest; and the fourth part with diseases of the
innermost parts of the chest and its contents; also with the arms
and hands. The fifth part will deal with affections of the body
in the regions situated between the chest and the genitals, the
sixth part being concerned with these latter. The seventh will
treat of all troubles from the anus downwards to the extremities
of both feet. Part eight will deal with abscesses; part nine with
wounds and all that pertains to them; part ten with fractures of
the bones; and part eleven with dislocations of the joints. In
part twelve we shall treat of simple, and in part thirteen of
compound, medicines. Part fourteen will be concerned with
laxatives and purgations for the noxious humours; whilst in
part fifteen will be found advice on phlebotomy, the regimen
of health, and many other things, as will appear later.

III. DE SIGNIS MALIS FEBRICITANTIUM ET ALIORUM INFIRMORUM

BREVIARIUM BARTHOLOMEI

PARS I, DISTINCTIO 6, CAPITULUM 19

Lambeth Palace Library MS. No. 444, f. 180.

Iste est paruus tractatus collectus ex dictis doctorum medicine de Signis pronosticis mortis. Et ponitur in speculo Johannis Mirfeld quod opus composuit in monasterio sancti Bartholomei Londonie iuxta Smyth-felde ac eciam aliud[1] opus composuit quod vocatur breuiarium bartholomei.

Cum accesseris ad infirmum primo memoriter attende considerando signa circà egrum aspiciendo eius vultum et linguam aperto ore. Et etiam oculi eius et vngues aspiciendi sunt et multa alia circa ipsum consideranda sunt vt in sequentibus manifestabitur[2]. Vnde scire debes quod signorum malorum apparencium in facie et oculis egrotantis quedam apparent infra iij primos dies et quedam apparent post. Illorum autem que apparent aliquando in primis tribus diebus sunt hec:—Oculi concaui: tympora plana: frons arida et tensa: nares acute: Aures frigide et inuerse et contracte; et color liuidus aut viridis aut niger et consimilia. Ista si ratione morbi proueniant in principio mortem signant potissime si egestio est liquida et vrina vnctuosa, sed non sic si apparuerint postea. Si vero ratione sinthomatum morbi talia appareant circa principium, Vt propter vigilias aut fluxum ventris aut famem et consimilia,

---

[1] *Sic* in MS.　　　　[2] "declarabitur" in Lambeth MS.

[1] "Other", *sic* in MS. The scribe evidently knew but has confused the two works of our author: the "Signs of Death" comes from the *Breviarium*. "Speculum" may refer to the *Breviarium*, the word being used in a loose sense (e.g. there is a medieval work entitled *Speculum Medicine*) in which case "Florarium" should be read for "Breviarium". It is quite likely, however, that the chapter as represented by the Lambeth MS. was inserted into a copy of

Plate 1

THE *BREVIARIUM BARTHOLOMEI*

Beginning of Chapter *De Signis Malis.*   Pars I, Dist. 6, Cap. 19

Harley MS, No. 3, f. 20

CONCERNING THE SIGNS OF EVIL PORTENT APPEARING IN FEVERISH AND OTHER TYPES OF PATIENTS

BREVIARIUM BARTHOLOMEI

PART I, DISTINCTION 6, CHAPTER 19

Rubric of Lambeth Palace Library MS. No. 444, f. 180.

This is a little treatise on the signs by means of which death may be foretold. It is compiled from the works of learned Doctors of Medicine, and is inserted in the *Speculum* written by John Mirfeld within the monastery of St Bartholomew, near Smithfield, in London; by whom also was composed that other[1] work which is known as the *Breviarium Bartholomei*.

When you visit your patient, you must bear in mind first of all the matters to which you should give heed, such as paying due regard to his countenance, and opening the mouth and looking at his tongue; moreover, his eyes and nails must be inspected, and consideration given to many other matters connected with him which will be set forth below. Wherefore, indeed, it should be known that of those signs of evil portent which manifest themselves in the eyes and features of the sick, some appear within the three first days of the onset of the disease, and others appear later.

Of such evil symptoms, those which sometimes appear within the first three days are these:[2] the eyes are hollowed, the temples sunken, the forehead dry and tense; the nostrils pinched; the ears cold, with the lobes turned outward and contracted; the colour livid, greenish or black, or something similar. If these symptoms appear at the commencement of the disease, and by reason of the virulence of the malady itself, then death is signified, especially if the stools be very loose and the urine oily: but this is not the case if they appear later. If however, the appearance of these signs in the opening stages is due, not to the severity of the disease itself, but rather to its accidents, such as sleeplessness, or frequency of stools, lack of

the *Florarium*, to which the title "Speculum" would more properly belong. Evidently the identity of authorship was known in the fifteenth century.

[2] The following passages are largely taken from a medieval Latin translation of the *Prognostics* of Hippocrates, perhaps that by Gerard of Cremona of the Arabic version of Hunain ibn Ishāk. For a direct translation from the Greek Text see that by W. H. S. Jones (William Heinemann, 1923, Loeb Classics), *Prognostic* II.

non est ita malum. Preterea si omnia ista predicta signa
propter morbum vltra tres dies apparuerint aut longe in
processu morbi, tunc non signant malum. Quia si in longo
tempore talia apparuerint, Non est mirabile nec signum
malum. Tamen intellige quod talia post principium ap-
parencia cum debilitate virtutis possunt signare mortem
licet non cum tanta efficacia sicut si apparuerint in principio. Quia rationabile est quod corpus infirmum per pro-
cessum temporis consumatur. Immo esset malum signum
si non consumeretur.

Signorum autem malorum que apparent in facie egrotantis quedam sunt que apparent post principium vt in
quarto die vel deinceps. Et sunt ista, videlicet:—quod infirmus non potest videre lumen candele et quod emittit
lacrimas inuoluntarias, et quod oculi appareant tornosi vt
alter altero minor fuerit. Vel quod albedo oculorum fuerit
sanguinea, et vene apparuerint nigre fusce aut pallide et
habeant lippitudinem et extra fuerint euntes aut intus
nimis existentes, et quod tota facies fuerit horribilis et tur-
pis aspectu. Ista, inquam, omnia signant mortem vt
plurimum. Et ista accidencia peiora sunt quam primo
dicta. Et etiam in principio possunt talia apparere; hoc
tamen est de raro contingentibus.

Possumus ergo concludere vt videtur quod quandocum-
que et vbicumque aut principio aut post ista omnia que
vltimo dicta sunt apparent propter morbi furiam et debilitatem virtutis mortem procul dubio signant. Et istis
predictis possumus alia signa addere mortalia, videlicet;—
si albedo oculorum in sompnis appareat, nihil tamen videat.
Et quod de saporibus nihil sentiat, Et quod consueuit sentire
et totaliter prohibeatur; Ita quod nihil odoret, Et appareant
dentes sicci sicut lingua. Ista et consimilia non solum signant mortem futuram sed mortem in ianuis. De talibus ergo
non te intromittas sed prognostica quod apparet, et recede.

food, and the like, then evil is not thus portended. Moreover, if all these aforesaid symptoms appear after the first three days, and result from the disease itself, or if they develope a good deal later during its course, then they are not of ill omen; because if they do not make an appearance until after a considerable lapse of time, then this is a matter neither of wonderment nor of concern. It must, however, be understood, that if such symptoms do appear after the commencement of the disease and accompanied by pronounced weakness, death may thus be signified, although not so effectually as when the appearance occurs at the beginning: for it is reasonable to assume that the body of the patient has been wasted away owing to the process of time; and it would, indeed, be a bad sign if such were not the case.

Of those signs of evil import, which appear in the features of the patient, there are some which show themselves later than the outset of the disease, such as on the fourth day or afterwards. They are as follows:[1] The patient cannot bear to gaze upon a lighted candle and he sheds involuntary tears, whilst the eyes appear to squint, and one seems smaller than the other: or the whites of the eyes appear bloodshot, and the veins black, swarthy, or sallow, the eyes inflamed, and the eyeballs protruding or sunken, whilst the whole aspect of the face is unsightly and horrible to look upon. These symptoms, I say, all signify death in most cases, and they are of worse import than those mentioned in the first place; they can also appear at the outset; but this, however, rarely happens.

We may therefore, it would seem, conclude that whenever and wherever, at the outset or later, all these last-mentioned symptoms appear on account of the fury of the disease and the weakness of the constitution, then most assuredly death is betokened. And to the aforesaid we may add some other indications of death; namely, if the whites of the patient's eyes appear during sleep,[2] without his being able to see anything; if he has lost all his sense of taste and is totally unable to discern those things, which he was once accustomed to perceive; and if he can smell nothing; and if the teeth also, as well as the tongue, appear dry. These and similar tokens portend not merely an approaching death, but death within the doors. With such cases therefore do not meddle. Let your prognosis be given, and then retire.

[1] Hippocrates, *Prognostic* II.　　　　[2] *Idem, Prognostic* II.

De hiis signis mortalibus habentur versus:

> Hiis signis moriens certis dinoscitur eger:
> Fronte rubet primo, pedibus frigescit ab imo,
> [1][Sponte sua plorans mortis pronunciat horam],
> Decidit et mentum nasus summotenus albet,
> Petrescit venter leuus minuetur ocellus.
> Excubeas patitur Iuuenis si nocte dieque
> Sique senex dormit designat morte resolui,
> [1][Aut si forte vadat in ventre virga virilis.
> Pluresis aut frenesis aut tertia sinocha causon
> Vrinas albas monstrantes hee moriuntur.
> Idropisi ptisi Apoplex paralisi dissinteria
> Vrinas rubeas monstrantes heu moriuntur.]

Preterea si infirmus iaceat resupinus pessimum signum est quia virtutis debilitatem signat. Similiter decubitus super ventrem est malum quia nimium dolorem signat vel alienacionem. Et si iaceat brachiis rigidis et pedibus malum est quia spasmus signatur. Et si post sompnum vel alias subito se vertat et inordinate vt a capite lecti vsque ad pedes alienacio et debilitas virtutis significatur. Et si iacuerit ore aperto et pedibus tortis malum quia spasmus. Et si subito cogatur surgere aut stare malum quia suffocacio propter stricturam viarum anelitus. Et si cum manibus festucas aut pilos aut consimilia temptet de vestimentis aut pariete remouere [laboret][1] potissime si ratio fuerit lesa sic quod non intelligat quid agat pessimum quia vltima adustio et mortificacio significatur. Item contractio labiorum aut manuum aut virge malum quia spasmus [in hoc significatur].[1] Item quia vngues ex cordis fumositatibus generantur,

---

[1] The words in brackets occur only in Lambeth MS. No. 444.

---

[1] *School of Salerno*, De Renzi, *Coll. Salernit.* Vol. I, p. 491, ll. 1400 *et seq.*
[2] See Hippocrates, *Aphorisms*, VII, lxxxiii: "When in illnesses tears flow voluntarily from the eyes it is a good sign, when involuntarily, a bad sign."
[3] These lines would appear to be based on the Hippocratic *Aphorism* VII, lxxii: "Both sleep and sleeplessness, when beyond due measure, constitute disease." See also *Aphorisms* II, iii.

Take note also of the following verses[1] indicative of a fatal termination:

When all these various symptoms in the patient do appear
Then you may safely prophesy that death at hand is near!
Dusky glows the brow, first the soles of the feet wax cold,
The dreadful hour of death is by the unwished tears foretold![2]
Downwards sags the chin; then pales to its tip the nose,
The belly rigid turns; the left pupil smaller grows.
Watch too for signs in sleep; for you can surely tell,
That Death doth strike a grey-beard who sleeps too sound and well,
Likewise the youth who night and day gains no repose at all,[3]
Or if perchance Priapism holds the sufferer in its thrall!
If white the urine be, when tertian, synocha, or causus[4] rages,
In pleurisy or phrenzy too, this death, alas, presages!
And when the sick be stricken with paralysis or dropsy,
With consumption, apoplexy, or with dysentery as well,
Then if the urine red appear of patients thus afflicted,
Alas, their plight is hopeless; you can merely death foretell!

Moreover, if the patient lies prostrate on his back, it is the worst possible sign, and indicates a vitality at its lowest ebb.[5] Likewise it is a bad sign to find the patient lying face downwards, for this indicates either excessive pain or delirium. And if he should lie with arms and feet rigid, this is an evil omen because it points to the presence of spasm. And if, after a sleep, or at other times, he suddenly turns himself about in a disorderly fashion, changing for example from the head to the foot of the bed, this shows delirium and bodily weakness; and if he lies stretched out with his mouth open and his feet twisted, this is grave, because it indicates spasm. And if he is suddenly constrained to rise up or to stand erect, this is grave, because it is due to suffocation arising from constriction of the respiratory passages. And if his hands are continually trying to pull straws or hairs, or the like, out of the bedclothes or from the wall[6]—especially if his reason be affected, so that he is unaware of what he is doing—then this is the worst possible sign, for it signifies the final consuming and mortification. Again, a drawing up of the lips, hands, or penis is bad, because this indicates spasm.[7] Also, since the nails are generated from the vapours coming forth from the heart, the vigour or

[4] "Synocha" and "causus" are continued fevers.
[5] See *Prognostic* III, upon which the following paragraph is based.
[6] This description of "Carphology" is taken from Hippocrates, *Prognostic* IV: "In acute fevers...if they (the arms) move before the face, hunt in the empty air, pluck nap from the bedclothes, pick up bits, and snatch chaff from the walls—all these signs are bad, in fact deadly."
[7] See Hippocrates, *Prognostic* IX: "Testicle or member being drawn up is a sign of pain or death."

cordis ipsius viuacitas vel mortificacio in eis apertissime
pronosticatur. Calore enim cordis deficiente vngues nigre-
scunt et pallescunt [vel liuescunt] Et ideo sui mutacione
vel contractione extraccionem caloris vel mortificacionem
nature presentant et pretendunt, vnde dicitur quod color
niger aut viridis in vnguibus cum aliis malis signis et ante
signa digestionis malum et mortale.

Item hanelitus frigidus et paruus aut magnus et frequens
aut cum sonitu in pectore malum et mortale. Cum autem
apparet in principio morbi vomitus niger mortem procul
dubio signat. Item omnis vomitus cuiuscumque condicionis fuerit dum tum venerit post signa digestionis et cum
alleuiacione pacientis bonus et laudabile quia venit per
viam mundificacionis; ideo nullus vomitus naturalis propter
quem fit alleuiacio debet restringi nisi excederet. Sed
vomitus sanguineus cum febre continua pessimum signum
est et etiam mortale. Item si vermes viui in principio morbi
in egestione apparuerint malum est quia signatur quod corrupcio tanta est quod vermes non possunt tollerare sed
fugiunt. Si vero mortui fuerint bonum est quia videtur
quod veniunt per viam mundificacionis: si autem in fine
morbi apparuerint mortui malum est quia ex malicia morbi
videntur esse mortificati; si viui bonum est quia ex mundificacione videntur prosilire. Item sudor superueniens febri-
citanti ante signa digestionis malum. Item sudor frigidus
si appareat in morbo acuto mortem signat: si in longo
longitudinem morbi signat.

Item Ictericia ante septimum[1] diem malum. Si post
septimum[1] diem si materia fuerit digesta et in die cretica[1]
semper est bonum potissime cum alleuiacione pacientis.
Item quando apparet apostema nigrum in summitate nasi

---

[1] Mirfeld seems uncertain in his use of the gender of "dies".

[1] "Digestio" in the Latin. We are obliged to Mr Fulton of the British
Museum for the information that the corresponding word in the Arabic text
is "Nudj", which has the meaning of "gestation", "maturity", and "ripe-
ness" (as applied to fruit, etc.), thus proving that the word "digestio" is a

decline of the latter organ may be ascertained most readily by an examination of the former of these members: for if the heat in the heart be insufficient, then the nails grow black, pale, or livid; so that by their change or contraction they present and show forth the withdrawal of the heat, and the departure of life. Wherefore it is said that a black or greenish colour in the nails, accompanied by other grave symptoms, and occurring before the signs of maturation, is an evil thing and denotes death.

Again, if the respiration be feeble and shallow, or if it be laboured and hurried, or accompanied by sounds within the chest, this is a bad symptom and points to death. When, however a black vomit appears at the beginning of a disease, most assuredly death is signified. All vomiting of whatever description, if it occur after the symptoms of the maturation of the disease, and which brings alleviation to the patient, is good and praiseworthy, since it comes as a cleansing agent; therefore any natural vomiting, which thus alleviates, should not be checked, unless it be excessive. Vomiting of blood, however, accompanied by continual fever, is the worst possible symptom, and is also mortal. Again, if live worms appear in the stools at the commencement of a disease, this is an evil symptom, because it signifies that the corruption of the body is so great that the worms have been unable to bear with it, and have taken to flight; if the worms be dead, then this is a good sign, because it would seem that their appearance is the result of a cleansing. If, however, the worms arrive dead at the close of the illness, then this is a grave matter, for they would seem to have been done to death by the malignity of the disease: if they be alive in such a case all is well, for they would seem to burst forth as a result of the cleansing of the patient. Again, perspiration supervening in a case of fever before the signs of maturation,[1] is of evil import; likewise death is portended by a cold sweat which appears in an acute disease: if it occur in a lengthy illness, it signifies that death is afar off.

Jaundice occurring before the seventh day is serious: but if it make an appearance after the seventh day,[2] and the bile be digested on the day of crisis, it is always of good import, especially when it brings relief to the patient. Again, when a blackish abscess appears suddenly on the tip of the nose,

translation of the Greek word πέψις. Mirfeld, following the Galenists, held that fever was produced by the presence in the body of morbid matter (the "materia peccans" of the Proemium), the expulsion of which, on maturity, constituted the crisis. "Digestio" was the stage during which the fever was ripening, and was terminated by the crisis.

[2] Hippocrates, *Aphorisms*, IV, lxiv.

subito cum forti dolore malum signum et mortale. Item
quando fuerint pustule nigre super digitos vtriusque manus
sicut orobus et dolor sit vehemens, moritur paciens in iiii⁰
die. Item fetor anelitus et oris in acutis egritudinibus signum est mortale. Item frequens in lecto reuolucio et ex
aliqua figura in aliquam diuersam mutacio malum. Item
quando eger super aliquod ex lateribus non quiescit sed
supinus iacere semper appetit Et preter hoc ad partem
pedis descenderit signum est mortale. [Item quando super
genu infirmi apparet pustula nigra vt vna nigra in cuius
circuitu sit nigredo mortale.]¹ Item alia accidencia ex
quibus homines verecundari consueuerunt vt cum aliquis
verenda discooperuerit vel cum ventositas inferius cum
sono egreditur significacio est non bona. Item squinancia
cum febre acutissima perniciosissima est.

Item oculorum stupor quorum palpebre non con-
iunguntur accidens est mortale. Item mortuorum nomina
proferre signum est malum. Quod si singultus fuerit secutus
erit perniciosum. Item cum oculus fit subito citrinus vel
niger aut eger prefocatur ita quod saliuam trahicere non
possit signum est perniciosum. Item cum in lingua apparuerint grana ciceribus in magnitudine equalia fueritque
febris acutissima eger in principio sequentis diei morietur.
Item secundum quod narrat Auicenna qui habet dolorem
hanche et apparet in coxa eius rubedo vehemens ad quantitatem trium digitorum non faciens ei dolorem et accidat
ei in ea pruritus vehemens et desiderat olera morietur in
xxvᵃ die. Item si infirmus frequenter respiciat manus suas
vel trahat pannos digitis vel manibus non est bonum signum. Item quando fuerit in vtroque genu infirmi apostema

¹ Sentence in square brackets occurs in Lambeth MS. only.

---

¹ At this point commences an extract from the "Signs of Evil Import in
Fevers" from Rhazes, *Liber Ad Regem Almansorem*, Lib. x, cap. 21.
² Much of this treatise on prognosis appears to be based upon haphazard
excerpts from the *Canon* of Avicenna, Lib. iv, Fen. 2, Tract. 1, C. 26 onwards.
³ At this point commences a series of extracts from the pseudo-Hippo-
cratic *Capsula Eburnea*, one of the spurious productions assigned to Hippo-

accompanied by considerable pain, then this is an evil sign, and is mortal. Again, when black blisters resembling the bitter vetch occur on the fingers of either hand accompanied by vehement pain, then the patient will die on the fourth day. Again,[1] foetor of the breath and mouth in acute diseases is a mortal sign. Again, frequent tossing about in bed, and changing from one posture into another, is an evil sign. Similarly, when the sick man can obtain no rest whilst lying upon either side but always desires to lie upon his back, and, moreover, slips down to the foot of the bed, then this is a mortal sign.

Another mortal sign is the appearance upon the patient's knee of a black pustule, that is, one with a blackish edging. Moreover, it is significant of evil when those actions which normally occasion embarrassment, such as the uncovering of the pudenda, or the audible expulsion of flatus from the bowel by the patient, occur (without perturbing him). Quinsy, again, with very acute fever, is most harmful.

Again, another symptom of death is when the eyes are dull and the eyelids not properly closed. Another sign of ill omen is the uttering by the patient of the names of those no longer living; and if hiccoughs follow, the result will be lamentable. Moreover, if the eye suddenly turns yellowish or black; or if the patient is choked so that he cannot swallow his saliva; then these symptoms are fateful. And when grains the size of a chick-pea appear on the tongue in conjunction with very acute fever, the patient will die at dawn on the following day.

Moreover, according to Avicenna,[2] when a patient feels pains in the region about the hip-joint, and then is affected with marked but painless erythema in that region extending over an area the size of three fingers, then if that spot begins to itch violently, so that the patient longs for the application of soothing oils, he will die on the twenty-fifth day. Again, it is not a good sign if the patient frequently looks at his hands, or claws at the bed-linen with his fingers or his hands. Again,[3] it should be

crates in order to give it currency, but perhaps Byzantine or even Arabic in origin. It derived its name from the account, with which it opens, of the supposed discovery of the original MS. within an ivory box placed in the tomb of Hippocrates. It was printed in the 1497 Latin edition of the works of Rhazes, but appeared frequently in manuscripts during the Middle Ages. We are indebted to Mr Fulton of the British Museum for the information that in the Arabic text (entitled 'Alāmāt al-ḳaḍāyā, or al-Rasā'il al-ḳabrīyah) it is ascribed to Hippocrates, who, feeling death near, ordered the twenty-five dicta to be set down in writing, placed in an ivory box, and buried with him; and that it was found by the Byzantine emperor who opened the tomb. According to the Arabic text, it was translated into Arabic from the Greek by Hunain ibn Isḥāḳ during the reign of the Caliph Ma'mūn (A.D. 813–833). The Arabic text was translated into Latin by Gerard of Cremona (1114–1187).

vehemens et magnum scias quidem morietur infra octauum diem et precipue quando in principio sue egritudinis suda-uerit sudore multo. Item quando fuerit in aliquo digi-torum pustula parua nigra sicut orobus et doleat tunc patiens morietur in secunda die Et signum illius est quod erit in egritudine sua grauis corporis. Item quando fuerit in police manus sinistre infirmi pustula parua fusci coloris vel pallidi que non dolet tunc scias quod morietur in vi[a] die sue egritudinis signum est quod in principio assellauit assellacionibus multis valde. Item quando fuerint vngues digitorum fusci coloris vel pallidi et in fronte pustula san-guinea tunc scias quod patiens morietur iv die. Et signum est quod multe erat sternutacionis et multe ocitacionis. Item quando fluit a naribus sanguis trahens ad subalbe-dinem, et apparet in manu dextera pustula alba non dolens, scias quod morietur die tercia sue egritudinis; signum est quod non desiderat cibum omnino. Item si eger in qualibet passione sudauerit a fine thoracis sursum fuge ab eo: si totus sudauerit bonum. Item qui habuerit febres quales vis si spasmum habuerit in illa febre scito eum mori.

Item quando fuerit sub ceruice pustula et in palpebra inferiori oculi sinistri pustula alia alba scias quod patiens morietur in xi die sue egritudinis. Et signum est quod accidit in principio egritudinis sue desiderium dulcium desiderio vehementi. Item si egrotus manus ad pedes flexerit nullo modo euadet. Item si egrotus insompnie-tatem passus fuerit et sepius ad hostium attenderit signat se recessum facere. Item in acutis infirmitatibus si videris stercus infirmi nigrum cum sanguine Et sine febri stercus nigrum aut vomitum nigrum, mortale. Item labiorum liuiditas signum est defectionis virtutis et caloris naturalis sicut econuerso rubedo labiorum signum est puritatis complexionis et interioris virtutis. Item sudores si frigidi facti fuerint in homine et semper concurrerint per faciem aut pectus curacionem significat. Item dicunt naturales

known that when a large and virulent abscess appears on either knee,[1] the patient will die within eight days, especially if he should perspire excessively at the commencement of his illness. Again, if there be on any one of the fingers a small black and painful blister similar in appearance to the bitter vetch, then the patient will die on the second day. And the symptom of that will be that he will be very much pained in his body during his illness. Again, when a small blister, dark or pallid in hue, appears on the thumb of the left hand without causing pain to the patient, then it should be known that death will ensue on the sixth day of his illness, and an indication of it is that at the commencement of his illness he went to stool profusely and frequently. Again, when the finger-nails are dark or pallid in colour, and a blood-coloured blister appears on the forehead, then know that the patient will die on the fourth day: and an indication is the occurrence of considerable sneezing and yawning. Again, when blood, rather pallid in colour, flows from the nostrils, and a painless white blister appears upon the right hand, then know that the patient will die on the third day of his illness; and the sign is that he has lost all desire for food. Again, if in any disease, the patient perspires from the base of the thorax upwards, flee from him: if he perspires all over his body it is well. Again, whosoever has fever, whatever you will, if he has spasm in that fever, then know that he will die.

Again, when there is a blister below the nape of the neck, and another white blister in the lower eyelid of the left eye, know that the patient will die on the eleventh day of his illness. And the indication of this is that at the beginning of his illness it happened that he most ardently desired sweet things.[2] Again, if the patient bends himself so that his hands touch his feet, then on no account can he escape.[3] Again, if the patient suffers from insomnia and somewhat frequently turns towards the door, it signifies that he will pass away. Moreover, in acute diseases if the faeces are seen to be black with blood, or even if without fever they are still black, or there be black vomit, then this is mortal. Again, lividity of the lips is a sign of the loss of strength and natural heat, just as, on the contrary, red lips show good health and internal strength.

Again, cold sweats in a man which drench the face or breast signify that a cure will take place. Again, natural philosophers say that those who are about to die, for three days

[1] "Both knees" in Arabic, according to Mr Fulton.
[2] End of *Capsula Eburnea* extracts.
[3] The "emprosthotonos" of tetanus described by Aretaeus.

easdem pupillas quas videmus in oculis per triduum mori-
turos non habere; quibus non visis certa desperacio est.
Item nudacio et inquietacio brachiorum mortiferum signum
in acutis est.

Item Auicenna dicit quod quando visitas infirmum si
tecum in manu tua portaueris veruenam et queras ab eo,
Quomodo est tibi? et si tunc ipse respondéat, Bene est
mihi, euadet. Si autem dixerit, Male, non euadet. Item
Experimentator dicit quod si Arthemesia[1] ponatur sub
capite pacientis ipso ignorante si dormierit viuet. Sin
autem, morietur.

Item si manus infirmi lineatur cum fermento et tunc
detur cani, si canis id comedat conualescet, si non morietur.

> Algor in extremis calor et sitis interiorum
> Hiis visis abeas: curam que geras aliorum.

Item, vngue diligenter totam plantam pedis dextri infirmi
de lardo et istud prohice cani. Et si hoc comedat et non
euomat viuet infirmus ille. Et si illud euomat vel non
comedat morietur. Item misce vrinam infirmi cum lacte
mulieris masculinum parientis. Et si misceantur inuicem
viuet, si non sed separatim permaneant morietur. Item
super viridem vrticam vrinam egri perfunde et alia die si
vrtica viridis permanserit viuet infirmus; si non morietur
adtunc. Item si oculus dexter hominis infirmi lacrimas
emittat pessimum signum est et mortale; et de femina
oculus sinister. Item si fiat emplastrum de musa enea et in
die non cretico ponatur super loca pulsuum si tunc patiens
sudauerit iudicandus est euadere. Sin autem nequiquam.

Item ℞ labdanum[2] et aloes, tere aloes, et confice cum
baldano[3] et fac inde candelam et appone morituro ad nares;

---

[1] Marginal note in Lambeth MS. "Mater herbarum".
[2] *Sic* in MSS. = λήδανον.   [3] *Sic* in *Brev.* MSS. for "labdano".

beforehand, lack natural pupils; and, if these be invisible, the case is certainly hopeless. Again, in acute diseases, uncovering and restlessness of the arms is a mortal sign.

Also, Avicenna advises the physician that, when he visits his patient, he should carry in his hand a twig of vervain and enquire of the patient, "How does this feel to you?" If he shall answer, "It is pleasant to me", then he will recover; but if, on the contrary, he shall say, "It is bad", then he will not escape. Also, the Experimenter[1] states that if, unknown to the patient, Artemisia (mugwort)[2] be placed underneath his head, then, if he shall sleep, he will live; if he do otherwise, he will die.

Again, if the hand of the patient be rubbed with yeast, and then this be offered to a dog, if the dog eats it, then the patient will be restored to health; if not, he will die.

Coldness of the extremities, thirst, heat in the inmost part,
Should'st thou perceive, retire thyself: to others take thine Art ![3]

Again, carefully anoint all over the sole of the patient's right foot with lard, and then throw the lard to a dog. If the dog eats it without vomiting then the patient will live, but if the dog returns it or makes no attempt to eat it, then the patient will die. Again, mix the patient's urine with the milk of a woman who has brought forth a male child: if the milk and urine mix well together, then the patient will live, but if on the contrary they remain separate, then he will die. Also, if the urine of the patient be poured over a green nettle, and if the nettle remain green on the next day, then the patient will live; if not, he will die very shortly.

Again, if the right eye of a sick man sheds tears, then this is the worst possible sign and is mortal: and in the case of a woman this applies to the left eye. Moreover, if a plaster be made from Musa Aenea[4] and this be applied to the places where the pulses are situated, on a day which is not a critical one, then if the patient shall perspire he can be judged as likely to escape. If otherwise, the labour is in vain.

Likewise take gum ladanum[5] and aloes, grind up the aloes and mix with the ladanum, and then make therewith a candle, and

---

[1] I.e. Rhazes.
[2] Marginal note in Lambeth MS. "Mother of Herbs".
[3] *School of Salerno*, De Renzi, ll. 2098, 2099.
[4] Musa Aenea is a "compound medicine" and a sedative, containing among other ingredients Opium and Henbane. The prescription is given in full in the *Breviarium*, Part XIII, Dist. 2.
[5] Resinous juice obtained from the lada shrub, *Cistus creticus*. (*Sinonoma Bartholomei*: "Lapdanum dicitur nasci de rore celi vnde dicitur quod lapdanum est ius coagulatum cadens super prunas et est calide et sicce complexionis.")

et quando calor tendit ad cerebrum aperiet oculos et tunc
pete ab eo quicquid volueris et dicet tibi, donec dicat, sine
memori.[1] Non probaui. Item si vis scire de aliquo vtrum
in breui sit febricitaturus faciat fleobotomiam in Maio vel
in Aprili et sanguine coagulato in vase superaspergatur sal
tostum. Si tunc post vnam horam sal feteat [in breui]
febricitet; si non, non.

Item quando minuitur quis accipe de eius sanguine
paruam quantitatem et mitte in calicem aque frigide
plenum et tunc ad fundum integre si descendat in ipso anno
non morietur; Et si se dissoluat et appareat quasi gutta
olei desuper periculum est.

Item si dubitas de aliquo an sit mortuus vel non appone
naribus eius cepam parum assam et si viuat statim scalpet
nares. Item si prima vocalis hominis monoculi vel mutulati
vel huiusmodi sit A vel O tunc patitur in parte dextera Et
si vocalis prima nominis eius sit E vel I vel V tunc patitur
in parte sinistra.[2]

At this point both the MSS. of the Breviarium *chapter finish:
the following continuation appears only in the Lambeth manuscript:*

Item, nudacio et inquietacio brachiorum mortiferum
signum est in acutis. Item quando spasmus euenerit post
laxatiuam acceptam signum mortis est.

Egritudinibus quibuscumque incipientibus si fel nigrum
aut sursum aut deorsum exierit mortale. Idropicus si
tussim habuerit mortale. Si videris egrotum frequenter
vertere se ad parietem malum est. Item si eger nihil
modicum[3] salutauerit malum est. Item si eger caput ad
pedes fecerit malum est et non euadet. Item Iusquiamum
tere cum succo mente et fronti inducas; si non dormierit
morietur. Item Vrinam infirmi pone in vno vase et facias
mulierem masculinum nutrientem ponere de lacte suo
iij guttas; si lac supernatauerit malum quia infra breue
morietur; et si lac misceatur cum vrina tunc euadet. In
muliere facias cum lacte mulieris feminam nutrientis. Item

---

[1] *Sic* in MSS. of *Breviarium*. In Lambeth MS. it runs "donec dimittat sui
memori".
[2] Marginal note in Pembroke College MS. "Credo in deum."
[3] *Sic.*? for "medicum".

place it to the nostrils of the dying patient; who, when he feels the heat penetrate through to his brain, will open his eyes: then ask him whatever you desire, and he will speak to you, whilst he retains consciousness. But of this I have not made proof.

Again, if it is desirable that it should be known whether a person will quickly become feverish, let phlebotomy be performed on him in May or April; allow the blood to coagulate in a dish, and then sprinkle roasted salt upon it: if, after an hour, the salt gives forth an unpleasant odour, the man is a feverish subject; otherwise not. Again, if your patient becomes thin, take a little of his blood and pour it into a cup full of cold water; if it all falls to the bottom in one mass, he will not die during the same year; but if it dissolves and appears, as it were, a drop of oil floating on the surface, then the patient is in danger.

Moreover, if there is any doubt as to whether a person is or is not dead, apply lightly roasted onion to his nostrils, and if he be alive, he will immediately scratch his nose.

Furthermore, if the first vowel of the name of a patient, who has lost an eye or is otherwise mutilated, be A or O, then he will suffer in his right side, and if it be E, I, or U, then in the left.[1]

*   *   *

Again, in acute diseases, uncovering of the body, and restlessness of the arms, is a deadly sign:[2] similarly when spasm follows the taking of a laxative.

If at the commencement of any illness whatever, black bile escapes either from the mouth or anus, this is mortal.[3] Dropsy accompanied by cough is fatal. It is a bad sign when the patient is seen to turn himself frequently to the wall; so also if he pays no attention to the physician. Again it is a bad symptom if he lies with his head touching his feet; nor can he recover.[4]

Again, grind up henbane with the juice of mint, and spread it over the forehead, and if the patient does not sleep, then he will die. Take also the patient's urine and pour it into a vessel, and then cause a woman, who is suckling a male child, to squeeze three drops of her milk into it; if the milk floats upon the surface it is of bad import, for within a short time the patient will die, but if the milk mixes with the urine, then he will recover. In the case of a female patient, make use of a woman suckling a female child.[5]

[1] At this point both MSS. of the *Breviarium* chapter end. What follows is in the Lambeth MS. only.
[2] Hippocrates, *Prognostic* IV.   [3] Hippocrates, *Aphorisms*, IV, xxii.
[4] The "emprosthotonos" sometimes seen in tetanus, described by Aretaeus.
[5] From the treatise on "Urines" by Johannes Afflacius (*circ.* A.D. 1040–1100), a pupil of Constantinus Africanus.

Accipe nomen infirmi et nomen nuntii et nomen diei qua
nuntius venit ad te, et coniunge omnium illorum litteras
simul; si numerus fuerit equalis non euadet, si impar
euadet. Item ista sunt signa mortis;—vomitus continuus,
sudor frigidus, frigiditas extremitatum, Multus singultus,
Spasmus parumquoque rationis, Omnimoda ventris con-
stipacio. Item si apparuerit pustula nigra super ventrem
sequente die morietur. Item si vultus pallido tumore
mictatus est virides oculi crurium tumor. Item si vene
circa oculos et in fronte nigre sint morietur. Ad id Accipe
herbam pentafilon[1] cum pater noster dicendo in nomine
egri colligatur, et coque hanc herbam in olla noua cum
aqua quam bibat patiens. Si aqua[2] sit rubea ex tali
decoccione viuet eger. Sin autem non. Quia morietur ex
tabellio Salerni in glosa.

Item, dixit Ypocras: Cum in sompnis apparet [apostema]
nigrum in posteriori aurium parte patiens morietur 7°[3]
die, et cum in iuncturis idropisis[4] exiuerit Apostema aut
in pede liberabitur post mensem a die quo apparuerit.

Super nasum autem si apparuerit pustula sicut pannus
lineus [mundus] aut nigra morietur in fine anni a die ap-
paricionis.

Et quando febriens habuerit dolorem sub ipocundriis
sinistris et apparuerit in loco Apostema et delicuerit subito
morietur in die 3°.[5]

Et si pustula nigri coloris in poplite sinistri pedis sit scias
quod pestilencia est; si patiens alienatus fuerit ante 3m diem
morietur ante viim diem.

Et si exitura pustule nigre in lingua fuerint febrientis in
die [non] cretico pronosticat mortem et signum est.

---

[1] I.e. "pentaphyllon".　　　　　　　[2] Sic in MS.
[3] Sic in MS.: for "xviijo".　　　　　[4] Sic in MS.: for "idropis".
[5] Sic in MS.: for "quarto".

[1] This is evidently inspired by a Byzantine version of the so-called "Sphere
of Pythagoras", a magical device which forecasts death by means of a series
of numbers arbitrarily placed in various positions within a circle, each number representing a letter of the alphabet, and the termination of the disease
being ascertained by the numerical value of the patient's name, and other
attributes. For further information thereon, see Dr Charles Singer, *From
Magic to Science* (1928).

[2] From this point onwards, until the lines from the *School of Salerno* which
end the treatise, the text consists of a verbatim copy of the greater part of the
Latin treatise on the signs of death which masqueraded during the Middle

Again, take the name of the patient, the name of the messenger sent to summon the Physician, and the name of the day upon which the messenger first came to you; join all their letters together, and if an even number result, the patient will not escape; if the number be odd, then he will recover.[1]

The following are the signs of death: Continuous vomiting, a cold sweat, and cold extremities, excessive eructations, convulsions and delirium, together with bowel obstruction of whatever nature.

Again, if a blister, black in colour, appear upon his belly, the patient will die on the following day; similarly, if the face be distorted with a pallid swelling, the eyes become greenish, or the legs swollen. Also the patient will die if the veins around the eyes and in the forehead appear black in colour.

Take the herb Cinquefoil, and, whilst collecting it, say a Paternoster on behalf of the patient, and then boil it in a new jar with some of the water which the patient is destined to drink; and if the water be red in colour after this boiling, then the patient will live; otherwise he will die, according to a gloss on the Salernitan Table.

Again, Hippocrates[2] said: when during sleep a black [swelling][3] appears behind the ears, the patient will die from the complaint on the seventh day;[4] and when in the joints or in the foot of a dropsical patient an abscess bursts, he will recover after a month from the date of its appearance. If, however, a pustule, the colour either of a [clean][3] linen rag, or black, makes its appearance upon the nose, the patient will die at the end of a year from the day of its first appearance. When a patient, stricken with fever, feels pain under the left hypochondrium, and an abscess appears in that region and suddenly disappears, he will die on the third day.[5]

And if there be a black blister on the popliteal space of the left limb, know that the pestilence is here; and if the patient be delirious before the third day, he will die before the seventh. If black blisters suppurate on the tongue of a feverish patient at a time which is [not][3] the day of crisis, this prognosticates and is

---

Ages under the name of Hippocrates, but which was probably Arabic in origin. It occurs in many medieval MSS., and was printed (together with the *Capsula Eburnea*, from which it is distinct) in the 1497 Latin edition of Rhazes, with the title "Gloriosissimi medici Ipocratis pronosticorum liber qui dicitur liber secretorum". The Lambeth transcript is often defective, inaccurate and almost illegible; consequently its variations from the generally accepted text have been indicated by means of footnotes.

[3] Hiatus in MS. Latin text. The authentic version is inserted.

[4] *Sic* in MS.: for "18th" of authentic text.

[5] *Sic* in MS.: for "4th" of authentic text.

Alienacio cito post dolor[em] totius corporis [et cardiaca statim post somnum] significat habundanciam humoris in corpore et pronosticat mortem subitaneam.

Cum exierit in palpebra patientis Apostema quasi Auellana sine dolore et grauitate morietur in iij mensibus.[1]

Dolor iuncturarum in iuuentute breuitatem vite significat. Cum in Ancha apparuerit apostema acutum morietur in iijbus mensibus. Qui patitur effimeram et fluxerit sanguis ab eius naribus morietur 30°[2] die.

Quando febriens manibus huc illuc quesierit et viderit mortuos morietur 15° die.

In cuius crure apparuerit pustula colore coleco[3] et flammens omnino morietur in mense primo. Et si fuerit sine ardore et pruritu morietur in sex[4] mensibus.

Pustule nigre et virides mortales maxime si fiant cum febre.

Item tortura mandibule vel obliquitas visus in febre acuta significat mortem statim.

Cuius oculi fuerint obliqui cito alienacionem significat.

Qui appetit commedere in horis non suetis humores in eius stomacho pronosticat: qui si fuerint sparsi [vel congregati] inferunt mortem.

Item qui loquitur subito turpia et appetit cibaria nociua debilitatem significat membrorum principalium.

Item iuuenis cui acciderit pleuresis magna morietur.

Cum acciderit febris cum tussi et subito tussis recesserit pronosticat apostema in aliqua iuncturarum.

In cuius corpore sepe acciderit dormitacio membrorum pronosticat ipsum mori subito propter paucitatem spirituum in corpore.

Qui piger est ad motum in ipso pronosticat dolorem iuncturarum.

Item cuius sudor acellarum fetet lepram pronosticat.

> Vnde dolet infirmus medicus sit pignore firmus;
> Instanter querere nummos vel pignus habere;
> Postea si queris tunc inimicus eris.

Amen. Explicit iste tractatulus multum necessarius.

---

[1] *Sic* in MS.: for "xxxiij° die".   [2] *Sic* in MS.: for "33°".
[3] *Sic* in MS.: probably for "colocasie".   [4] *Sic* in MS.: for "septem".

a sign of death. Delirium following quickly upon pain affecting the whole body, [and heartburn immediately after sleep],[1] signifies an excess of humour in the body, and portends sudden death. When an abscess having the appearance of a filbert nut breaks out upon the eyelid, unaccompanied by pain or heaviness, the patient will die in three months.[2] Pain in the joints of the young signifies a brief life.[3] When an acute abscess breaks out in the region about the hip-joint, death will occur within three months. Whoever suffers from ephemeral[4] fever, accompanied by bleeding from the nose, will die upon the thirtieth[5] day. When a fever-stricken patient fumbles hither and thither with his hands[6] and in his delirium sees friends no longer living, he will die upon the fifteenth day. Whoever has an acutely inflamed blister the colour of an Egyptian bean[7] upon the leg, will die during the first month; and if it occur without heat and itching, he will die in six[8] months. Black and greenish blisters are fatal, particularly when they appear in association with fever. Also, twisting of the jaws or squinting, in acute fever, portends immediate death; and squinting signifies delirium soon to come. Whenever a patient desires food at unaccustomed times it points to the existence of humours in his stomach, which, if they spread [or gather together],[1] will cause death; and whenever he suddenly says shameful things and desires harmful foods it indicates a failure of the higher centres.

A young man who falls into a serious attack of pleurisy will die. When fever is accompanied by cough, and the cough suddenly disappears, it points to an abscess in one of the joints. Whoever suffers from frequent numbness of the limbs will, one can foretell, die suddenly from the lack of vital spirits in his body; one can also prognosticate that the man who is averse to taking exercise will have pain in his joints; also that offensive perspiration from the armpits betokens "leprosy".[9]

> [10]Whilst groan the sick with pain, the doctor must be sure
> To pocket his reward, or gain a pledge secure.
> Whoever this defers until the patient's health shall mend,
> Demanding then his fee, doth lose the name of friend.

Amen. Here endeth this very necessary little tract.

[1] Hiatus in MS. Latin text. The authentic version is inserted.
[2] *Sic* in MS. for "33rd day" of authentic text.
[3] Does this perhaps refer to rheumatism in the young leading to valvular disease, and thus to early death?
[4] An ephemeral fever was regarded as arising from a "dyscrasia of the spirits". It usually lasted for twenty-four hours and terminated in sweating.
[5] *Sic* in MS. for "33rd" of authentic text.
[6] Carphology. Hippocrates, *Prognostic* IV.   [7] Colocasia.
[8] *Sic* in MS. for "7" of authentic text.
[9] "Leprosy" at this date included many varieties of skin disease.
[10] *School of Salerno*, De Renzi, ll. 2086 *et seq.*

IV. DE PTISI

BREVIARIUM BARTHOLOMEI

PARS IV, DISTINCTIO I, CAPITULUM 13

Non te lateat quod ptisis quandoque large quandoque
stricte accipiatur; large vt in senibus qui consumpti sunt
ex etate, et vt in pacientibus febre acutissima vt dictum est
superius parte prima. Stricte autem accipiatur vt quando
ex vicio pulmonis fit, et sic diffinitur. Ptisis est consumpcio
totius corporis ex vlceracione pulmonis de qua hic trac-
tatur. Contingit enim quandoque quod ex empimate cadit
patiens in ptisim vnde pulmo bibit humiditatem corporis
nutrimentalem Ideo extenuatur corpus et multo educit
per os de eadem humiditate.

Hoc modo perpenditur de aliquo vtrum sit ptisicus vel
non. Si ptisicus est, continue febricitat, sed calor febris
parum distat a naturali. Calor tamen sentitur in cute et
tabescit totum corpus et vngues habent in medio eleuatos,[1]
et sputum fetidum si ponatur super carbones viuos. Et si
in nocte sputum eius in pelui recipiatur et in mane aqua
calida super infundatur apparebit in superficie aque quedam crassities, in fundo putredine remanente. Et in fine
morbi cadunt capilli, fluxus enim ventris vel capillorum in
ptisicis mortem proximam notat.

Multi enim decipiuntur in cognicione ptisicorum, quosdam enim iudicant ptisicos cum non sunt. Ad cuius rei
probacionem magister meus tale faciebat experimentum.

----

[1] *Sic* in MSS.: add "et lateraliter curvos".

----

[1] Hippocrates, *Aphorisms*, v, xv: "When empyema follows on pleurisy,
should the lungs clear up within forty days from the breaking, the illness
ends; otherwise the disease passes into consumption."

[2] Hippocrates, *Aphorisms*, v, xi: "In patients troubled with consumption,
should the sputa they cough up have a strong smell when poured over hot
coals, and should the hair fall off from the head, it is a fatal symptom."

Plate II

THE *BREVIARIUM BARTHOLOMEI*

First portion of the Chapter *De Ptisi*.   Pars IV, Dist. I, Cap.13

Harley MS, No. 3, f. 88

Reproduced by courtesy of the Trustees of the British Museum

ON PHTHISIS

BREVIARIUM BARTHOLOMEI

PART IV, DISTINCTION I, CHAPTER 13

It should be observed that the word "Phthisis" is capable both of general and of special application, for it is sometimes used as a general term to denote the wasting away due to advanced age, or to that resulting from acute fever, as has been explained already in Part I of this compilation: its use, however, should strictly be confined to that form of wasting which is provoked by some disease of the lungs, and it is in this restricted sense that it forms the subject of these pages, and is defined as follows: "Phthisis is a wasting away (a "consumption") of the whole body arising from ulceration of the lung." It does, indeed, sometimes happen that a patient falls into consumption after an attack of empyema,[1] when the lung drinks up the health-giving moisture of the body, so that much of this moisture drains away through the mouth, and emaciation results.

The following is the method by which it may be determined whether a patient is phthisical or not. If phthisical there will be continued feverishness, but the height of the fever will be a little only above the normal. The heat is felt, however, in the skin, and the whole body dwindles away; the nails become elevated in the middle [and curved at the sides]. The sputum also gives a foetid odour if dropped upon live charcoal.[2]

If also the patient's sputum be collected in a basin during the night and hot water be poured upon it in the morning, the solid parts will appear floating on the surface of the water, whilst the putrefying matter remains at the bottom.[3]

As the end approaches the hair falls out; and indeed looseness of the bowels or loss of hair portends that the death of the phthisical patient is near at hand.[4]

[5]Many practitioners are led astray when dealing with this disease, for they diagnose many as suffering from consumption who are not really so affected. The following is the test which

---

[3] The whole of the text up to this point is a verbatim extract from the *Practica* of Magister Bartholomaeus of Salerno (*flor. circ.* A.D. 1100).

[4] Hippocrates, *Aphorisms*, v, xii: "Consumptive patients, whose hair falls off from the head, are attacked by diarrhoea and die"; see also *Aphorisms*, v, xiv.

[5] The next two paragraphs are copied verbatim from the *De Causis, Signis, et Curis Egritudinum* of Magister Johannes [II] Platearius (*flor. circ.* A.D. 1100).

Ore enim aperto faciebat egrum hanelare, et cum hane-
litum eius sentiret corruptum et valde fetidum ita tamen
quod tempore sanitatis hanelitus eius non fuisset fetidus
ptisicum illum iudicabat et incurabilem.

Item ptisicus in volis manuum et plantis pedum habet
calorem continuum secundum maius et minus. Et sitim
patitur cum asperitate lingue et palati et cum colli gracili-
tate et totius corporis macilencia; ventris patitur consti-
pacionem et extremitatum vnguium constriccionem et
orbium oculorum concauitatem. Familiare autem signum
est dolor sinistre spatule vsque ad humeros.

Preterea sciendum est quod differentia est inter ptisim
et ethicam quia in ethica pulmo non est lesus et habens
eam non habet tussim. In ptisi autem est pulmo lesus et
habens eam non autem est sine tussi. Item differentia
est inter sputum saniosum et sputum fleumaticum, quia
sputum saniosum quando submergitur in aqua petit fundum; fleumaticum vero supernatat; et discernantur iterum
fetore quia sputum saniosum quando spergitur aut quando
prohicitur super carbones fetet, fleumaticum vero non.

Vlterius sciendum est quod si hec passio cadat in
fleumatico et humido extendi potest vsque ad xx vel xxx
annos; si in melancolico et sicco vel in colerico non ita
durabit et est curabilis.

Item, in ptisi fetor oris preter solito est signum mortale,
et si sputum fuerit saniosum et fetidum, et cum hoc adest
casus capillorum et diarria, mortem signat.

Preterea cauendum est diligenter in pronosticacione
ptisicorum quia interdum loquendo moriuntur et moriendo

---

¹ "My Master." The authentic Platearius text gives "Pater meus", i.e.
"My Father" (i.e. John Platearius the Elder). Mirfeld has altered this into
"My Master" just as he has done when quoting Lanfranc of Milan (see
Introduction, pp. 10, 23). Does he merely mean to infer that he himself has
taken Platearius and Lanfranc as "masters", or does he really intend to
imply that he studied under a master who used as his text-books the writings
of these authors? This latter proposition would seem to conflict with what
he himself says in his preface, viz. that he never was a pupil.

My Master[1] used to apply: He made his patient open the mouth and exhale: if he perceived the sick man's breath to be foul and strongly foetid, whereas this had not been the case when the patient was in good health, then My Master[1] pronounced him to be suffering from phthisis and incurable.

Again, the consumptive suffers more or less from continual heat in the palms of the hands and the soles of the feet; from thirst accompanied with dryness of the tongue and of the palate, and thinness of the neck together with leanness of the whole body. He is also troubled with constipation, constriction of the tips of the nails, and hollowing of the eyeballs. A familiar sign, too, is pain in the left shoulder-blade reaching as far as the shoulders.

Moreover, the difference between consumption and hectic fever should be realised; for in the latter disease the lung is not damaged and the patient has no cough, whereas in consumption there is an injury to the lung, and the patient is not without a cough. There is also a difference between sputum which contains blood and simple phlegm, for the former kind of sputum when dropped into water falls to the bottom, whereas the latter floats on the surface; they may, moreover, be distinguished by the odour, for the sanguineous sputum, when it is smeared or dropped upon glowing charcoal, smells evilly, whereas phlegm does not.

[2] Finally, it ought to be known that should this disease attack one of phlegmatic and moist temperament, it may be prolonged for twenty or thirty years; if, however, the patient be melancholic and dry, or choleric, then the complaint will not run so long a course, and is curable.

Likewise abnormal foetor of the breath is a morbid sign in phthisis: and if the sputum should become blood-stained or foetid, and this be accompanied by falling out of the hair, and by diarrhoea, this also betokens death.

Moreover, great caution must be exercised in making a prognosis in cases of consumption, for sometimes whilst speaking these patients die, and whilst dying they converse.

Again, consumptives become more oppressed, and their symptoms aggravated, after taking food; their cheeks become flushed, and they sometimes feel pain in the middle of the neck.

---

[2] From this point onwards, the rest of the text (with the exception of some of the prescriptions) consists almost entirely of a series of literal quotations (strung together, however, without any regard to the correct arrangement) from the chapter on "Phthisis" in the *Lilium Medicine* of Bernardus de Gordonio, which itself incorporates Hippocrates, the *Methodus Medendi* of Galen, and the *Canon* of Avicenna.

loquuntur. Item ptisici magis laborant et aggrauantur post cibum quam ante. Et cum hoc habent rubedinem in maxillis et aliquando dolor adest in medio colli.

Item, si vlcus fuerit in pulmone tunc multum leditur patiens a quocumque aere excedente siue calido siue frigido. Et non potest patiens iacere in aliquo laterum et dolor est in mamilla sinistra. Item, ptisici aliquando expellunt tussiendo partem pulmonis aliquando partem venarum et aliquando lapidem.

Item si pustula appareat super spatulas moritur infra lij dies. Et vlcus saniosum pulmonis non recipit curacionem propter causarum contrarietatem vt enim vlcus mundificetur oportet vt tussis prouocetur vt per tussim purgetur sanies, sed tussis et concussio magis augmentant vulnus et ideo incurabile. Signa autem quibus testantur ptisicum morti approximaturum sunt casus capillorum, incuruacio vnguium, prostracio appetitus, difficultas hanelitus, retencio sputi, fluxus ventris, inflacio tibiarum. Et vt plurimum ptisici expediuntur cum folia cadunt ab arboribus, Autumpnus enim detegit ptisicos quia in autumpno manifestatur. In ptisico fluxus ventris casusque pilorum, Faciesque rubens sputi fetor sunt signa periculi. Istis signis non apparentibus ptisis potest longo tempore palliari in pueris et senibus et pinguibus et carnosis.

Item, ptisis adolescentulis vel iuuenibus citra quadragesimum annum superueniens multum in antea[1] non protenditur, sed primo anno aut soluitur aut interficit.

Cura enim ptisicis est secundum duas res quarum vna est vera et altera blandiens. Cura quidem vera est quando egritudo est curabilis et est cum mundificacione vlceris et siccacione ipsius et prohibicione catarri et expulsione materie a pulmone. Blandiens vero est quando egritudo non est curabilis.

Et intelligendum est quod in ptisi sunt tria, scilicet, vlcus, sanies, et consumpcio. Vlcus indiget consolidatiuis, sanies mundificatiuis, et consumpcio nutrientibus et re-

---

[1] *Sic* in MSS.: for the "ultra annum" of Platearius, from whom this sentence is taken.

If there be ulceration of the lung, then the patient is much harmed by exposure to abnormal atmospheric conditions, whether heat or cold; nor can he lie on either of his sides, and he is troubled with pain in the left breast. Sometimes, too, consumptives during bouts of coughing spit up part of their lungs, sometimes part of their veins, and sometimes even a stone.[1]

Again, if a pustule should appear on the shoulder-blades, the patient will die within fifty-two days.[2] An ulcer of the lung associated with haemorrhage does not lend itself to cure on account of the contrariety of the factors at work: for, in order to cleanse the ulcer, it is necessary to provoke coughing, so that the corrupted blood may be purged away by means of the cough; but since the coughing, and the shaking resulting therefrom, only make the wound worse, it is therefore incurable.

The signs, however, by which the approaching death of consumptives may be known, are as follows: Falling out of the hair, incurving of the nails, distaste for all food, difficulty of respiration, retention of sputum, diarrhoea, and swelling of the lower limbs. Most cases of consumption develope when the leaves fall from the trees; indeed, autumn is the great detector of consumptives, for it is then that this disease is made manifest.[3] In consumption, frequency of stools, loss of hair, a flushed countenance, and foetid sputum are signs of danger, but, if these symptoms are not apparent, then the progress of the disease can be stayed for a long time in the case of children, elderly people, and those who are plump and well-nourished.

Again, a consumption which attacks adolescents or persons under forty years of age does not last for longer than one year, for within this time it is either cured or else it kills the patient.

There are two types of *treatment* for consumption, namely, the complete cure and the palliative. The complete cure is naturally only possible where the disease is curable, and it consists in cleansing and drying up the ulcer, together with the prevention of catarrh, and the expulsion of matter from the lung. The palliative treatment refers of course to the incurable cases.

Now it must be realised that in phthisis three factors require consideration: the ulceration of the lung, the corrupt blood-stained matter contained therein, and the wasting away of the patient. The ulcer needs consolidative medicines, the corrup-

[1] The second of these refers no doubt to the blood-casts of the bronchial tubes sometimes coughed up in haemoptysis: the last to the "pneumoliths" or small calcified portions of tubercle which consumptives occasionally spit up.
[2] B. de Gordonio ascribes this to Avicenna.
[3] Hippocrates, *Aphorisms*, III, x: "Autumn is bad for consumptives."

sumptiuis. Nunc autem deus creauit vnam medicinam vbi
sunt ista tria, scilicet, lac. In lacte enim est natura cerosa,
propter quam abstergit, et ibi est natura caseata, propter
quam consolidat. Est etiam ibi natura butirosa, propter
quam nutrit et reparat. Ideo summe competit lac et precipue lac mulieris, deinde asine, deinde capri. Modus
autem sumendi sit ab vbere. Et si non est possibile,
habeatur scutella abluta cum aqua calida et stet super
aliam plenam aqua calida et mulgeatur et exhibeatur
statim quia lac citissime corrumpitur. Et si timemus cor-
rupcionem bulliat ad ignem et ponatur ibi modicum salis
et mellis et sorbeatur, aut prohiciantur in lacte lapides
fluuiales candentes, aut ferrum candens. Et in toto illo
tempore quo lac est in stomacho non debet sumi vinum,
quoniam vinum facit lac coagulari in stomacho. Et cum
coagulatum est iam transit in naturam veneni. Item,
vinum competit ptisicis, quoniam abstergit, et mundificat,
et nutrit, et velociter conuertitur in calorem et spiritum: sit
ergo vinum album quodammodo dulce et debile vel sit
vinum citrinum clarum cum multa aqua ordei vel pluuiali.

Item ptisana ordei prodest multum; abstergit enim et
mundificat et nutrit et infrigidat. Et potest dari in ptisi,
siue detur lac siue non, et siue sit febris siue non: sed
cauendum est a lacte similiter et a vino cum adest febris
putrida. Et potest ptisana dari ante cibum et post cibum,
et tam in nocte quam in die, seruata quantitate debita.
Similiter et mel multum prodest ptisicis, quoniam abstergit et mundificat, et nutrit, et penetrat; Et ideo est
vehiculum omnium medicinarum que valent ad spiritualia.

Si autem adest febris fetida aut calor fortis, posset tem-
perari, et dari ydromel aquaticum cum zuccaro multo.

---

[1] Is this an early indication of pasteurisation, to prevent the milk turning
sour?

[2] Hippocrates in his *Regimen in Acute Diseases*, Lib. i, regards "white" wine as
in general the best, saying, "it always is in many ways beneficial in acute diseases", though "sweet wines" and "astringent dark wines" also have their uses.

[3] *Ibid.* Many sections of the *Regimen*, from par. x onwards, deal with the
proper preparation and due administration of barley-water and barley-gruel
in acute diseases.

tion requires cleansing, and the wasting restorative and nourishing medicines. Now, however, God has created one single medicine, namely *Milk*, which contains these three attributes; for in milk there is found the expulsive power of wax, the consolidative properties of cheese, and the nourishing and reparative qualities of butter. Therefore milk is of the greatest possible value, especially if it be that of women; asses' milk is next to be preferred, and then that of goats. The milk ought to be imbibed direct from the udder; but should this be impossible, then take a salver, which has been washed in hot water, and allow it to stand over another full of hot water; then let the animal be milked into the salver and the milk immediately proffered, for it very quickly turns bad.[1] If it be feared that this has occurred, boil the milk over the fire, add a pinch of salt or honey to it, and let this be absorbed; or drop into the milk either heated stones taken from the river, or a red-hot iron. Moreover, wine should not be drunk during the whole period in which the milk remains in the stomach, for the wine causes the milk to coagulate, and this changes it into the nature of a poison.

Wine agrees with consumptives, for it drives away what is harmful, it cleanses and nourishes, and is quickly turned into heat and life-giving spirit. Let the wine, however, be white,[2] somewhat sweet, and weak, or let it be clear and golden in colour, and taken with plenty of barley-water or rain-water.

Moreover *barley-water*[3] is a very beneficial drink, for it possesses expulsive properties, is cleansing, nourishing, and cooling; and it can be given in cases of phthisis irrespective of whether milk is, or is not, taken; nor need any question be raised as to the presence of fever: but the physician must be guarded in prescribing milk[4] or wine in cases where there is putrid fever. Barley-water may be given before or after meals, and either by day or by night, provided that the correct quantity be taken.

Similarly *honey* is very beneficial to consumptives, for it expels, cleanses, nourishes, and penetrates, so that it is the vehicle for all medicines which are beneficial to the "spiritual members";[5] but, where the patient is afflicted with a foetid or high fever, it is wise to temporise and administer the honey in the weaker form of Hydromel Aquaticum,[6] with plenty of sugar.

[4] Mirfeld here probably has in mind the Hippocratic dictum: "Milk is beneficial in cases of consumption when there is no very high fever" (*Aphorisms*, v, lxiv).

[5] The "spiritual members" are the heart, lungs, etc.

[6] Honey, and especially Hydromel (honey-water), are also recommended in acute diseases by Hippocrates, who says: "Hydromel...softens the lungs, is mildly expectorant, and relieves a cough" (*Regimen in Acute Diseases*, Lib. III). *Sinonoma Bartholomei*: "Idromel...multociens tamen sumitur pro mulsa."

Item cancer fluuialis est cibus altissimus in isto casu et medicina beata. Decoquatur ergo in aqua dulci donec possit mundari Et abiectis exterioribus interiora et extremitates fortissime abluantur cum lexiua[1] facta de aqua cinerum vitium deinde decoquatur ad perfectionem cum aqua ordei Et comedatur substancia et aqua decoctionis potetur.

Item zuccara rosarum multum prodest de qua dicit Auicenna. Ego, inquit, sum multociens expertus in corporibus diuersis et in regionibus diuersis, quod multum confert ptisicis zuccara rosarum recens si vtantur ea spacio vnius anni omni die quantum potuerit patiens quamuis multum sit: vnde vt dicit Auicenna, Funeralia erant parata cuidam mulieri ptisice et frater suus curauit eam cum multitudine accepcionis zuccare rosarum; sed tanta fuit quantitas quod quasi incredibile est. Et si constringatur hanelitus patientis propter exsiccaccionem rosarum, detur ei in potu syropi papaueris albi ℥ſs post zuccaram rosarum. Et non intermittatur hec cura quoniam sanat.

Item ficus sicce perutiles sunt, similiter et vue vsuales mundate ab arillis, similiter et nuclei pinearum et huiusmodi. Et potest comedere carnes omnium [auium] volatilium, vsualium preter quam de illis que degunt in aquis. Potest enim vti carnibus edinis mutouinis et vituli lactantis vel cuniculi iuuenis et extremitatibus animalium vt sunt pedes et crura porcellorum et galline et pulli earum et caro annualis agni. Et de omnibus istis parum et raro preter quam de volatilibus et de illis accipiat in tam parua quantitate quod possit digeri. Et vtatur testiculis vulpis et pulmone eiusdem quia mirabiliter competunt. Et vtatur lacte amigdalarum et amidi.

Et interdum potest vti spinarchiis boraginibus et feniculo, petroselino, et portulacis. Et potest vti piscibus squamosis de aquis mundis currentibus et ouis sorbilibus. Detur

---

[1] *Sic* in MSS. for "lixiuio".

The *River-crab* is the finest possible food for use in this disease, and is indeed a blessed medicine. It should be boiled down in sweet water until it has been cleansed. Throw away then the outside parts, and thoroughly wash the insides and the extremities with lye made from the ashes of burnt vines mixed with water; then let it be cooked to perfection in barley-water, whereupon the flesh may then be eaten, and the water in which it has been boiled may be drunk.

Another very efficacious medicine is *Sugar of Roses*, concerning which Avicenna[1] speaks as follows: "I, myself, have often proved, both on different patients and in various places, that freshly-made Sugar of Roses is very beneficial to consumptives, if daily for a whole year as much of it be administered as the patient can take, even although the quantity be great." Wherefore, as Avicenna[1] says, "the funeral rites of a certain consumptive woman were made ready, but her brother cured her by dosing her plentifully with Sugar of Roses, so much, indeed, as almost to be incredible". And if the patient's breathing be embarrassed on account of the dryness produced by the Roses, then administer half an ounce of Syrup of White Poppy in his drink,[2] after he has partaken of the Sugar of Roses. And do not relinquish this treatment, for it cures.

Again, dry figs are very useful and so too are the ordinary kinds of grapes when the pips have been removed: moreover pineapple kernels, and foods of that nature, are beneficial.

The patient can also eat the flesh of all the usual kinds of fowl which fly, except of those which live on the water; likewise the flesh of kids, lambs, and unweaned calves, or of the young rabbit; also the extremities of animals (such as the feet and legs of little pigs), hens and their chickens, and the flesh of a year-old lamb: and of all these only a little should be taken, and but rarely, except in the case of flying fowl, and even this should be taken only in such a small quantity as to be digestible. Also the patient may use the testicles and lung of the fox, for these are marvellously beneficial. Likewise milk of almonds and starch[3] may be employed with advantage.

Occasional use may be made of spinach, borage, fennel, rock-parsley, and purslane; also of fish covered with scales if taken from clear running water; also of eggs which can be

[1] *Canon*, Lib. III, Fen. 10, Tract. 5, Cap. 6.
[2] This prescription is here given in preference to that of Avicenna and of B. de Gordonio, who give "Syrup made from hyssop and lozenges of camphor or gum tragacanth".
[3] *Sinonoma Bartholomei*: amidum=amilum.

etiam ei interdum musa cum succo liquiritie et dragaganti et vitet acetosa salsa et acuta.

Item cibus confortans. ℞ farine frumenti rizi ana li .i. Ista decoquantur in brodio galline et collatura detur. Item brodium decoctionis arietine carnis iuuatiuum est et nutrit ptisicos vt ait Haly. Item si pira aut poma deco-quuntur in aqua de illis potest comederi aliter non.

Item mundificacioni est gargarismus iste in quo omnes auctores conueniunt. Accipe cancros fluuiales et decoqu-antur sub cineribus donec caro resoluatur et tunc extra-hatur caro et iterum decoquatur in aqua cum ordeo excortitato. Et tunc exprimatur fortiter inter duos baculos per pannum. Et cum ista decoctione fiat frequens vsus gargarismi et aliquid de ipso transgluciatur.

In cura huius infirmitatis extrahatur aqua a floribus yreos ad modum aque rosarum. Deinde tere rosas et misce cum predicta aqua et sic stent per diem naturalem deinde coletur et de colatura illa in sero recipiatur. Et postea in mane iste sequentes pillule teneantur sub lingua que valent contra asperitatem gutturis et tussim et prohibent catarrum et faciunt dormire. ℞ tyriace magne ℨ iii succi liquiritie, seminis papaueris albi, dragaganti, gummi arabici ana ℨ ii opii Ɔ i. Conficiantur pillule cum succo papaueris albi et de nocte teneat duas sub lingua quousque dissoluantur.

Item electuarium ptisicorum ℞ Piperis albi, zinziberis ana ℨ ii, castorei, leuistici, ana ℨ i et semisse; maratri, semi-nis petroselini amei¹ ana ℨ semisse mellis quantum sufficiat.

---

¹ *Sic* in MSS. = ἄμμι.

¹ "Musa" is the "Muzi" or "Mauzi" of Avicenna (*Canon*, Lib. ii, Tract. ii, Cap. 492), i.e. Mauz, the fruit of the plantain or banana (*Musa Paradi-siaca*).

² This is all from the *Canon* of Avicenna but much abridged (Lib. iii, Fen. 10, Tract. 5, Cap. 6).

³ Iris Florentina. *Sinonoma Bartholomei*: "Yris purpureum florem (in modum azuri) gerit yreos album." Its root is orris-root.

⁴ "Tyriac" or "theriaca" (lit. "antidote") was a panacea, the invention of which was attributed to Mithridates, King of Pontus, which contained

sucked. Also, let the patient now and again be given banana[1]
with the juice of liquorice and of gum-tragacanth, and let
him shun things which are bitter, salt, and sharp.[2]

Another strengthening food: Take a pound each of the flour of
corn and rice; boil them up together in chicken's broth, and let
the repast be taken. Again, according to Hali Abbas, broth
made from boiled ram's-flesh is very helpful in nourishing consumptives. Moreover, if apples or pears be first boiled in
water, they may be eaten; otherwise not.

Furthermore, the following *gargle* is good for cleansing purposes, as all the authorities agree: Take River-crabs and boil
them beneath ashes until the flesh becomes soft. Then extract
the flesh, and boil again in water containing barley stripped of
the husks. Then, with the aid of two sticks, squeeze out forcibly
through a cloth. Make frequent use of this as a gargle and let
some of it be swallowed.

Another method of treating this disease is with a watery extract
of the flowers of the White Iris[3] made in a manner similar to
that followed in the preparation of rose-water. Then crush some
roses and mix them with the aqua, and allow the preparation
to stand for the duration of an average day, after which strain
and let the infusion be taken in the evening. Next morning
let the following *pills* be held under the tongue, for they are
useful against soreness of the throat and cough, and prevent
catarrh and induce sleep: Take of Great Tyriac[4] three
drachms; of juice of liquorice, of white poppy seed, of gum-
tragacanth, and of gum-arabic, of each two drachms, and of
opium one scruple. Make into pills with the juice of white
poppy, and at night keep two under the tongue until they be
dissolved.

Likewise an *electuary*[5] for consumptives: Take of white
pepper and of ginger each two ounces; of castoreum[6] and
lovage of each one ounce and a half; of fennel, rock-parsley
seed, and bishop-weed, of each half an ounce; and of honey as
much as shall suffice. Moreover this electuary for use in con-

originally thirty-eight, and later many more, ingredients, including opium,
and was held in high esteem until the eighteenth century A.D. It was
regularly taken as a preventive of disease; but was valued chiefly as an
antidote to poisons on account of the viper's flesh which formed one of its
ingredients (and to which it owed its name) being considered, according to
the theories then held, to be an efficacious cure for snake bites.

[5] An electuary is a powder made up into a paste with honey or syrup, etc.

[6] Castoreum is an animal product obtained from the beaver in a manner
somewhat similar to the musk obtained from the preputial glands of the
musk deer. *Breviarium Bartholomei*, Part XII: "Castor est testiculus cuiusdam
animalis quod dicitur castor siue beuer."

Item ad restaurandum humiditatem ptisicis et consumptis valet electuarium ptisicorum.

Item vnguentum de adepibus valet ptisicis si inde vngatur pectus vel vngue pectus cum butiro recenti aut cum oleo amigdalarum dulci vel cum dialtea et cum oleo violarum vel cum pinguedine porcorum vel cum auxungia anatis vel caponis. Et superpone pellem agninam. Et in crastino absterge cum colatura furfuris. Istud est inquit apud me summum experimentum in ptisi et ethica et in consumptis et in tussientibus.

Item balneum ad idem probatur; accipiantur catuli ceci et extrahantur viscera et abscindantur extremitates postea decoquantur in aqua et in ista aqua balneetur patiens. Et intret istud balneum post cibum per iiii horas et cum fuerit in balneo teneat capud coopertum. Et pectus teneat inuolutum cum pelle eduli ne pectus possit subito infrigidari.

Aliud balneum ad idem expertum. Accipe de testudinibus nemorum et decoquantur in cacabo. Et in prima vnda accipiantur testudines et extrahantur medulle et carnes et decoquantur in secunda aqua et in illa aqua balneetur patiens et post balneum inungatur pectus cum vnguento ptisicorum[1] vel alio predictorum. Et spina dorsi et vole manuum et plante peduum et iuncturalia inungantur cum vnguento isto. ℞ olei violarum olei rosarum olei nemiferis ana ℥ iii misceantur.

Si autem paciatur fluxum ventris restringatur pro posse quia citissime duceret eum ad mortem. ℞ ypoquistidos,

---

[1] *Breviarium Bartholomei*, Pars xiii, distinctio 7, capitulum 52: "*Vnguentum ptisicorum* sic fit. ℞ dragaganti albi gummi arabici ana ℥ ii adipis anseris anatis et galline ana ℥ iij medulle bouine cerui et vituli butiri recentis auxungie porci cere albe olei violarum ana li ſs. Terantur et liquificiant in patella ad ignem et simul decoquantur et incorporentur. Deinde depone ab igne et predictis appone puluerem dragaganti et gummi arabici et bene misceantur cera alba iuncta et fiat vnguentum. Et quando vti volueris tepefiat et inde inungatur spina dorsi et spondilia vsque ad inferius. Et ita in parte anteriori. Et scias quod multum confert hoc vnguentum contra ethicam et ptisim et tussim ex siccissitate."

sumption is of value for restoring humidity to phthisical patients and to those who are wasting away.

Again, an *unguent* made from the fat of animals is beneficial to phthisical patients, if the chest be anointed therewith. Other useful chest-ointments are those made from fresh butter, oil of sweet almonds, marsh-mallow root, or oil of violets; likewise one made from the fat of pigs, or grease made from ducks or capons. And over these place a lamb's skin. Then on the following day wipe away the ointment with strained bran. "This", he says,[1] "has been proved very efficacious by me in consumption, in hectic fever, in consumptive patients, and in those afflicted with cough."

Also here is a *bath* which has been proved to be of value. Take blind puppies, remove the viscera, and cut off the extremities; then boil in water, and in this water let the patient be bathed: let him enter the bath for four hours after his food, and whilst therein keep the head entirely covered, and the chest completely wrapped around with the skin of a small kid, as a preservation against exposure to sudden chill.

Another bath of which the patient may avail himself: Take land-tortoises, and boil them in a cooking-pot. Take the tortoises, whilst in this water, and extract the innermost parts and the flesh; then boil them in fresh water, and in this water let the patient bathe; and after the bath anoint the chest with either the "ointment for consumptives",[2] or with one of the others mentioned above. Anoint moreover with the following unguent the back-bone, the palms of the hands, the soles of the feet, and the joints: Take of the oil of violets, the oil of roses, and the oil of water-lilies, of each three ounces, and mix together.

If the patient be afflicted with diarrhoea, let this be restrained as much as possible, for very quickly it brings him to

---

[1] I.e. John of Gaddesden in the *Rosa Anglica*, Chap. *De Ptisi*, from which this paragraph is taken.

[2] *Breviarium Bartholomei*, Part XIII, distinction 7, chapter 52: "*The Ointment for Consumptives is thus made*: ℞ of white gum-tragacanth, of gum-arabic, of each two ounces; of the fat of geese, ducks, and hens, of each three ounces; of the innermost parts of the bull, stag, and calf, of fresh butter, of grease made from pigs, of white wax, oil of violets, of each half a pound. Let them be taken and liquefied in a pan over the fire and boiled down together into one substance. Then remove from the fire and add to the aforesaid some powdered gum-tragacanth and gum-arabic, and let them be well mixed together, having added some white wax: and make an unguent.

And when it is desired to make use of the ointment warm it gently, and then anoint with it the spine and vertebrae to the base thereof. And so too with the front part of the chest. And know that this unguent is of great benefit in hectic fever, consumption, and dry cough."

88   'BREVIARIUM BARTHOLOMEI'

acacie, sandali rubei, spodii, kakabre, gummi arabici assi, dragaganti assi, mirtillorum, sumacis ana ℨ ij, liquiritie mundate, caricarum, vuarum passarum, pinearum, ana ℨ semisse, conficiantur cum syropo mirtino et fiant trocissi. Et cum vti volueris distemperentur in lacte vbi fuerit ferrum ignitum et extinctum et ita restringetur; vel sic ad idem, In predicto lacte ponatur puluis sanguinis draconis aut boli armenici. Tamen si febrem fortiter habeat non vtatur lacte.

---

¹ Solidified juice of the *Cytinus hypocistis*. (*Sinonoma Bartholomei*: "Ipoquistidos est succus fungi qui nascitur ad pedem rose canine.")

² "Spodium" is soot from metal furnaces. *Sinonoma Bartholomei*: "Spodium quidam dicunt esse ebur combustum quid nihil est sed Spodium est fuligo que inuenitur in domibus vbi funduntur metalla que postquam ceciderit dicitur esse spodium...Nos tamen vtimur pro eo ebore combusto vel quod melius est loco eius cinere qui inuenitur supra fornaces argentariorum, lauatur autem vt ferrugo."

Plate III

THE *BREVIARIUM BARTHOLOMEI*
Second and concluding portion of the Chapter *De Ptisi*
Pars IV, Dist. 1, Cap. 13.   Harley MS, No. 3, f. 88 b
Reproduced by courtesy of the Trustees of the British Museum

his death. Take hypocistis,[1] acacia, red sandal-wood, spodium,[2] amber[3], roasted gum-arabic, roasted gum-tragacanth, myrtles, sumach, of each two drachms; of clean liquorice, dried figs, sun-dried grapes, pineapple kernels, of each half a drachm. Let them be prepared with syrup of myrtle, and made into lozenges. And when it is desired to make use of them temper them with milk in which a red-hot iron has been quenched; and thus the flux can be restrained; or for the same purpose put powdered dragon's-blood[4] or "Bolus armeniacus"[5] into the aforesaid milk. If, however, the patient has a raging fever, do not make use of the milk.[6]

[3] *Sinonoma Bartholomei*: "Cacabre vulgo dicitur lambra".
[4] "Sanguis draconis" is a resin obtained from the fruit of the *Calamus draco*: it is an astringent.
[5] "Bolus armeniacus" is also an astringent: it is a yellow earth containing iron oxide.
[6] Hippocrates, *Aphorisms*, v, lxiv.

V. PULVIS PRO INSTRUMENTO BELLICO

BREVIARIUM BARTHOLOMEI

PARS XIII, DISTINCTIO 4, CAPITULUM 12

Pulvis pro instrumento illo bellico siue diabolico quod vulgariter dicitur gunne.[1]

Accipe salis petre pondus xx d redige in puluerem subtilem. Item accipe sulfuris vi pondus x d. Item accipe salicem et combure et cum bene fuerit ignita claude in olla vel in alio vase ne fumus possit exire et ibi permittatur vsque fuerit extinctus ignis per se. Accipe de illis carbonibus pondus xij d et fac inde puluerem. Et misce ista tria predicta Et tunc habes puluerem conuenientem ad hoc opus et ad multa alia. Vel sic secundum quosdam debet proporcionari. ℞ salis petre pondus xvj d et obolus sulfuris vj pondus xiij d et obolus de carbonibus salicis vel sarmentorum vitis pondus iiij d et ob. Misceantur et vtere ad predicta. Vel sic. Accipe salis petre pondus xix d et ob. sulfuris vi pondus xj d et ob. carbonorum salicis pondus vij d et ob.

VI. EMPLASTRUM BARTHOLOMEI

BREVIARIUM BARTHOLOMEI

PARS XIII, DISTINCTIO 8, CAPITULUM 9

Emplastrum hoc valet ad omnes plagas siue capitis siue corporis et etiam ad cancrum et fistulam mortificat. Et sic potest fieri. Accipe succum apii, plantaginis et bulliant simul. Et cum bullire inceperint apponatur subtilis farina frumenti et bene moueatur vltra ignem donec incipiat inspissari. Et in fine decoctionis apponatur mel ad quantitatem aliorum et simul decoquuntur ad spissitudinem emplastri. Et vsui reseruetur.

[1] "gonne" in Harley MS. No. 3.

GUNPOWDER

BREVIARIUM BARTHOLOMEI

PART XIII, DISTINCTION 4, CHAPTER 12

Powder for that devilish instrument of war colloquially termed gunne.[1]

Take one pound and twenty pennyweights of saltpetre and reduce it to a fine powder: also six pounds and ten pennyweights of sulphur: also take willow wood and set fire to it, and when it is well alight enclose it in a pot or in some other such vessel so as to prevent the smoke from escaping, and let it remain thus until the fire has burned itself out. Of the charcoal thus obtained take one pound twelve pennyweights and make thereof a powder. Then mix these three aforesaid ingredients together, and then you have a powder suitable for the required purpose and for many others moreover.

Or thus, according to some people, ought the ingredients to be proportioned: Take of saltpetre one pound sixteen and a half pennyweights, of sulphur six pounds thirteen and a half pennyweights, of charcoals made from willow wood or vine twigs one pound four and a half pennyweights. Mix together and use for the purposes aforesaid.

Or thus: Take of saltpetre one pound nineteen and a half pennyweights, of sulphur six pounds eleven and a half pennyweights, of willow wood charcoal one pound seven and a half pennyweights.

THE PLASTER OF BARTHOLOMEW

BREVIARIUM BARTHOLOMEI

PART XIII, DISTINCTION 8, CHAPTER 9

This plaster is valuable in all wounds, whether of the head or of the body, and it also cures both ulcer and fistula. And it can be made thus: Take the juice of the parsley and the plantain and bring them to the boil together: and when they begin to boil add some fine corn flour, stirring well over the fire until thickening results. At the finish of this decoction add honey in a quantity equal to that of the other ingredients, and then boil them all down together until the consistency of a plaster is reached. And reserve for use.

[1] "gonne" in Harley MS. No. 3.

VII. "INCIPIT DE PONDERIBUS ET MENSURIS"

BREVIARIUM BARTHOLOMEI

Pembroke College, Oxford, MS. No. 2, f. 349 *b*

Oportet modo pondera medicaminum mensurasque eorundem cognoscere. Intellige ergo secundum doctrinam auctorum quod xx grana frumenti faciunt ℈i. Et ℈iii faciunt ʒi. Sed in pecunia nostra non possumus accipere pondus certum. Tamen apotecarii ponunt denarium pro ℈i, sed ℈i non ponderat denarium sed iii quadrantes cum tercia parte vnius quadrantis. Quia ℈iii faciunt ʒi Et ʒi ponderat iid. et obolus. Et ʒi cum dimidio facit solidum exagium et aureum que tria idem sunt in pondere licet nomina diuersificentur. Et secundum doctrinam antiquorum ʒix faciunt ℥i Et ℥12 libram i. Et libre ii cum dimidio faciunt sextarium i.

Sed nostri apotecarii qui emunt ad vnam mensuram et vendunt ad aliam habent vt dicitur libre ii, scilicet libra magna et libra minima. Libra magna ponderat xxvi s. et viii d sterlingorum: Et habet ℥ 16. Sed libra parua non ponderat nisi xx s. sterlingorum et habet ℥ 12. Et sic ℥ ponderat xx d. sterlingorum. Et x denarii faciunt ʒiiii. Apotecarii autem ponunt pro ℈i denarium i; Et pro ʒi ponunt iid et obolus; Et ℈iii ponunt pro ʒi; Et pro solido ponunt ʒi et semisse. Et per libram magnam deberent venderi omnia liquida scilicet syrupos olera et huiusmodi. Et per libram minorem omnia sicca vt zinziber gariofili et huiusmodi.

ON WEIGHTS AND MEASURES[1]

BREVIARIUM BARTHOLOMEI

Pembroke College, Oxford, MS. No. 2, f. 349 b

It is now necessary to become acquainted with the weights of the medicines to be used, as well as with their measurements. Understand that according to the doctrine of standard authors, twenty grains of corn make one scruple, and three scruples make one drachm. Owing, however, to our coinage system one cannot with accuracy make use of the above scale: nevertheless, our apothecaries use a penny to represent a scruple, although one scruple is not equivalent in weight to a penny but only to three farthings plus the third part of a farthing. Now because three scruples make one drachm, therefore one drachm is equal in weight to two pence and one halfpenny. Also one drachm together with half a drachm is equivalent to a solidus, hexagium, or an aureus, which three are the same in weight although their names are different. According to the doctrine of the ancients also, nine drachms make one ounce, and twelve ounces one pound, and two and a half pounds one sextarius.

But our apothecaries who buy according to one scale and sell according to another, use, as it is said, two different pounds, namely the large pound and the small pound. The large pound is equivalent in weight to twenty-six shillings and eight pence sterling, and consists of sixteen ounces. The small pound, however, weighs only twenty shillings sterling and contains only twelve ounces. Therefore an ounce is equivalent in weight to twenty pence sterling; and ten pennies make four drachms. The apothecaries, however, use a penny for a scruple, two pence halfpenny for a drachm; and they use three scruples for one drachm, whilst instead of one shilling they use one and a half drachms. The large pound is used for selling all liquids, for instance, syrups, oils, and the like: whilst the small pound is used for all dry goods such as ginger, cloves, and matters of that nature.

[1] This extract is of interest in showing the early use by the Apothecaries of the two measures: *Troy* or *Apothecaries'* (12 ounces to the pound) for weighing dry drugs, *Avoirdupois* (16 ounces to the pound) for weighing liquids. This has long, however, been superseded, and to-day all drugs, whether solid or liquid, are sold by avoirdupois weight. The habitual use at this date of the scruple, a weight now rarely used, is also interesting.

[Eight lines from the *Schola Salernitana* (...including "Constat sex solidis vel ter tribus vncia dragmis...".)]

Ex predictis patet quod secundum vsum modernorum ϑ ponderat id ℥ iii scrupulos siue iij d.

Solidum ⎫
Exagium ⎬ ℥ j et ſs.
Aureum ⎭

Obolus pars vjᵃ ℥ et ponderat 12 grana ordei i ℥ ponderat ℥ viij secundum quosdam xx d libra constat ex 12 ℥....

...Quarta anglicana li. ij continet.

VIII. EPILOGUE

BREVIARIUM BARTHOLOMEI

Hic autem compilacionis huius facio finem gratias agens ei cuius magnitudinis non est finis. Protestor autem in fine huius opusculi quemadmodum et in principio quod de omnibus que in hoc tractaculo continentur nichil quod est ad propositum de meo apposui quia quod apponerem ex meipso in meipso non inueni. Sed simpliciter philosophorum et phisicorum autenticorum verba et practicorum sententias collegi et collectas conscripsi in summula vna vt simplices et pauperes copiam librorum non habentes in promptu hic valeant inuenire saltem superficialiter plurimorum egritudinum remedia non pauca. Quod cedat oro ad proximorum vtilitatem et ad ipsius precipue honorem et gloriam qui est alpha et ω principium et finis omnium bonorum qui est deus benedictus sublimis et gloriosus viuens et regnans in secula seculorum. Amen.

[Then follow eight lines from the *School of Salerno* on Weights and Measures, comprising in versified form the theory ascribed by Mirfeld to the "ancients", i.e. that nine drachms make an ounce. He then continues as follows:]

It is apparent therefore, from what has been said above, that according to the usage of the moderns,[1] one scruple weighs one penny, a drachm is equal in weight to three scruples or three pence. The solidus, hexagium, and aureus, weigh one and a half drachms. The obolus is the sixth part of a drachm and is equal in weight to that of twelve grains of barley. And according to this method of calculation the ounce is equal in weight to eight drachms or twenty pence. Twelve ounces make a pound.

...An English quarter contains two pounds.

[1] I.e. the English system.

EPILOGUE

BREVIARIUM BARTHOLOMEI

I here make an end of this my compilation, and in so doing I give thanks unto Him of whose greatness there is no end. I protest, however, at the finish of this little work, just as I also did at the beginning thereof, that with regard to all the things which are contained in this little tract, I myself have added nothing of my own to the matter in hand, for the reason that I have not discovered anything of my very own to add. I have simply collected the words of authoritative philosophers and scientists, as well as the opinions of practical men, and having collected them together, have written them all down in one little summary: so that poor and unlearned men who do not possess a plenty of books at hand may here be able to find, at least in superficial degree, not a few remedies for very many diseases. And I pray that this book may prove of assistance to my neighbours and above all to the honour and glory of Him who is Alpha and Omega, the Beginning and the End of all goodness, who is God, blessed, glorious, and sublime, living and reigning for ever and ever! Amen.

§ III
The Florarium Bartholomei

III

THE *FLORARIUM BARTHOLOMEI*

I. INTRODUCTORY REMARKS

THE *FLORARIUM BARTHOLOMEI* of John de Mirfeld is not a medical, but a theological book which
consists of a Prologue, Epilogue, and 175 chapters,
and contains one chapter (lxxxviii) entitled "Physicians and
their Medicines". The work has survived only in imperfect
manuscript copies, of which several have been traced in old
library catalogues and ten (including fragments) found still
to be extant.

The author's original manuscript, however, has been
lost, and no more than two copies of the complete work
are available, viz. MS. No. 4 in Gray's Inn Library and
Royal MS. 7. F. XI in the British Museum: moreover,
neither is free from corruptions and obvious misreadings of
the original exemplar. It is therefore impossible to be certain whether the text compiled by collating the various
manuscripts in fact faithfully represents Mirfeld's own
words, nor can any accurate deductions be made concerning the learning of our author, when no certainty
exists as to whether he himself was responsible for the
numerous unintelligent misquotations from standard books
which appear in his compilation.

It is evident that the *Florarium* was not utterly ignored
or despised in Mirfeld's day: for the number of copies and
abstracts that were made would seem to indicate that the
work was fairly well known and appreciated: in the case of
Harley MS. No. 106 it was obviously considered of sufficient
importance to ensure that extracts from it should be bound

up with tracts by such important writers as Richard Hol-croft and John Bromyard.

Nor does the identity of the author appear to have been a secret, for, in spite of his attempt to suppress it by the adoption of the title *Florarium Bartholomei* for his work, as explained in the Preface, and the concealment of his name from the uninitiated by means of the acrostic, to some, at least, of his contemporaries, his name was known. Thus the abstract of the first half of the *Florarium* which is found on folio 129 of Harley MS. No. 106, and which was certainly written during Mirfeld's lifetime, is prefaced by the following sentence:

Nota hic quedam secundum quod habentur in florario bartholomei, quem librum compilauit Johannes de Mirfelde Johanni de Suthwelle

which distinctly states that John de Mirfeld compiled the book for John de Suthwell.

The name of the compiler seems, however, to have been soon lost to sight. Leland does not mention either the *Florarium* or its author, although he refers to "Marfeldus" as a medical writer; whilst Bale, Pits, and Tanner, in their collections of English literary biographies, follow Leland in considering Mirfeld to be a writer only of medical books, and they refer to the author of the *Florarium* as a separate person under the name of "Bartholomaeus Florarius", and describe him as a man who died about A.D. 1420.

The true identity of the compiler of the *Florarium* con-tinued to be wrapped in obscurity until the publication, in 1869, of A. J. Horwood's *A Catalogue of the Ancient Manu-scripts belonging to the Honourable Society of Gray's Inn.* Horwood, when describing the copy of the *Florarium* (MS. No. 4), pointed out that after the colophon following the end of the text there occurs a Latin couplet:

Ad Ihc incipias Capitales, non Aliunde;
Tunc quo vado scias, venio tibi lector et Vnde.

This is followed, in a smaller and different handwriting to that of the manuscript, by:

> Ad ihc accipies capitales et inde notabis
> Tunc quo vado scies venio simul vnde probabis.[1]

Having followed out the injunction contained in these verses, Horwood found that chapter lxii ("De hoc nomine Ihesus") was the one which opened with the word "IHESUS"[2] (I.H̄.C.), and that, on writing down the initial letter (I) of this and of each of the succeeding chapters of the work, the following sentence was obtained:

> *Iohanni de Suthuuelle per Iohannem de Mirfeld: Ora pro nobis beate Bartholomee vt digni efficiamur promissionibus Cristi. Amen. Explicit.*

This sentence, which may be freely translated as "Written for John de Suthwell by John de Mirfeld: Pray for us, O Blessed Bartholomew, that we may be made worthy of the promises of Christ. Amen. The end", would seem to leave no doubt as to the authorship of the work. It remained only for Sir Norman Moore to show that a similar acrostic runs through the *Breviarium Bartholomei*[3] for the connection between the two books to be demonstrated, and the identity of authorship to be established.

A final and not too valuable confirmation of such identity (if confirmation be needed) is provided by the inferences to be drawn from the wording of the fifteenth-century rubric to the Lambeth Palace MS. No. 444, f. 180,[4] as well as by the similarity of the literary style (such as it is) and the

---

[1] The second of these two couplets occurs also at the commencement of the preface to the Sion College copy (except that "incipies" is used instead of "accipies"). As a footnote to f. 3 of the British Museum MS. 7. F. XI the lines appear in this form:

> "Ad Ihs incipies capitales inde notabis
> Nunc quo vado scies, venio simul vnde probabis."

[2] It actually commences "Ihesus interpretatur Saluator".

[3] I.e. "Ora pro nobis sancte Bartholomee ait Iohannes dde Mirfeld vt digni efficiamur promissionibus Cristi, etc." (see p. 40).

[4] See p. 54.

tone in which the two books are written and the similarity of their conception as revealed in the prefaces.

The *Breviarium* is written in order to serve as a useful compendium to those who are too poor to afford the large number of medical books necessary to acquire the knowledge requisite for the preservation of bodily health, and to prevent such persons from falling into the hands of avaricious physicians. The *Florarium* on the other hand is intended as a similar guide to the attainment of spiritual health, and to prevent mankind from falling into the snares of the Evil One. Too much stress need not, however, be laid on this point, for it was a common habit amongst medieval writers to seek for some such pious excuse with which to preface and to justify their publications.

The question which next presents itself is that of the identity of the man to whom the book is dedicated. He was presumably the John de Suthewelle the "King's Clerk" who on the 19th of October 1382 obtained a royal letter to the sheriffs of London[1] directing the payment to him of an annuity of £10 out of the issues or farm of London which the king had confirmed on the 11th of March 1378, and which had originally been granted him for "good service" by Edward III on the 10th of November 1362[2] in lieu of a surrendered grant of ten marks yearly dated the 10th of June 1360.[3] He also seems to have been a Proctor in the Ecclesiastical Court at York, acting sometimes as Official to the Archbishop. In his youth he would naturally have been familiarly acquainted with his Chancery colleague, the elder William de Mirfeld: and it is therefore not difficult to imagine that he was thus introduced to John our author, who perhaps dedicated the work to him as the last survivor of William's contemporaries. If he is indeed the

[1] *Calendar of Close Rolls*, 1381–1385, p. 160.
[2] *Calendar of Patent Rolls*, 1361–1364, p. 266.
[3] *Calendar of Patent Rolls*, 1358–1361, p. 374.

individual to whom the *Florarium* was dedicated, then the reference in the Preface to "certamina curialium", the strifes of the Courtiers, would be satisfactorily explained.

The date of composition of the *Florarium* cannot be stated with any degree of certainty, except that it is obviously later than the year 1362, since Simon Islip's *Constitutions*, to which Walsingham has ascribed that date, are quoted in it; and probably also after 1369, since in it there is a reference to a sermon of "John Cronson" i.e. John Grandison, Bishop of Exeter (1328–1369), which would probably have been cited in a somewhat different form had the bishop been still alive.

At the end of the excerpts from the *Florarium* in the Sion College manuscript (f. 164 b) occur some verses followed by the sentence:

M. cum quater. C. Anno domini simul. X. et. Primo namque die Mensis Julij sibi cesset. Anno domini Millesimo. cccc^{mo}xl^{o}vij^{o}. Amen quod Johannes Hebyn, Diaconus.

From this it would appear that Deacon John Hebyn copied out the manuscript in 1447, and that he considered that the *Florarium* itself was originally finished on the 1st of July 1410. It has already been shown that John Mirfeld died in 1407, so that on this ground the ascription of the date 1410 would appear incorrect. It is now tentatively suggested that John Hebyn, when copying out the Sion College manuscript, may have actually transcribed from an earlier copy of the *Florarium* containing the first part of the colophon just quoted, and that he made the very natural error of confusing the sign $\mathcal{X}$ which was the usual medieval method of representing the Arabic numeral 4, with a very cursively written Roman "x" ($\mathcal{X}$) which would be very similar in appearance: thus one arrives at the date 1404. As John Mirfeld was ordained priest in 1395, and died in 1407, and as in his Epilogue he refers to the "little of life" that remains to him, it is quite possible that the year 1404 saw the completion of the *Florarium*. More especially would this seem to be the case when it is realised that at approximately that date John de Suthwell ceases to appear in the Patent Rolls as charged with legal commissions on behalf of the Crown; and that on the 28th of February 1405 he obtained the ratification of his estate as prebendary of Howden in Howden collegiate church,[1] in contemplation perhaps of that approaching retirement to which reference is made in the introductory dedication to him.

The *Florarium*, as has already been stated, is not a medical, but a theological book; and it seems, in effect, to be what is known as a "speculum", or "mirror", a species of compilation which was in great favour during the time in which Mirfeld lived.[2] Although the term "speculum" was often applied to any form of summary, it generally denoted a collection of theological tracts, usually on the cardinal virtues and vices, and embellished with illustrations, such as Mirfeld's story of the dying physician, which were intended to drive home a moral lesson. These books were generally arranged on a system which permitted the speedy finding of a reference, rather than the logical exposition of a pre-determined hypothesis. Such is the scheme of the *Florarium*, which was written, as the compiler says, in order to be a readily accessible guide to every department of the Christian life; and it is therefore arranged alphabetically according to the Latin name of the subject of each of the 175 chapters, every one of which is, as he himself says, quite self-contained, and capable of being treated as a separate entity.[3] Such a method of compilation was quite usual at this period, and is that employed by Mirfeld's famous contemporary, John Bromyard, in his *Summa*

---

[1] *Calendar of Patent Rolls*, 1401–1405, p. 451.
[2] E.g. The *Speculum Laicorum, Liber Exemplorum, Speculum Sacerdotis*, and many others. [3] See p. 164.

Predicantium. What apparently differentiates Mirfeld from his contemporaries is the inclusion of the chapter on Physicians; and the amount of space which is devoted to this subject shows that it must have been very near to his heart. Apart, however, from the inclusion of this particular chapter, there is but little differentiation between the *Florarium* and similar compilations. In his deference to accepted authority, as we may see from his Prologue and from the work itself, Mirfeld is at one with his contemporaries, although, whilst a priest himself, he does not hesitate to attack his colleagues the "spiritual physicians".

It is true that he lived in the time of Wycliffe, when the medieval theories of Church and State were being challenged, but he himself had no desire to come into conflict with the ruling powers. His age was indeed one which, if it did not discourage originality and experiment, nevertheless imposed upon the original genius the necessity of convincing his fellows that he was doing no more than bringing forward what had always been accepted by their fathers. Consequently we should not expect to find, nor indeed do we find, anything in the *Florarium* (especially in a chapter on a scientific subject such as Medicine), which would be in any way at variance with the accepted authority of the day, or which contains anything new or provocative in the way of medical advice.

As an examination will disclose, the whole of the medical section of the chapter is copied almost word for word from other writers of accepted authority. The only additions thereto—as for example those concerning the English method of taking food, and the recommendation of a particular brand of wine—occur merely as explanatory notes to make the work more readily comprehensible to an English reader. This is the method generally followed in medieval medical composition, and is typical of the age in which it is written. Herein, however, lies the special interest of this chapter of the *Florarium*, since it shows not only the nature of the general advice for the maintenance of health that would be given by a man living at the end of the fourteenth century, who had written so complicated a prescription book as the *Breviarium Bartholomei*, but also the type of reading, and the names of the authorities upon which this advice is based. Moreover, this identical advice is contained also in that part of the *Breviarium* itself which is devoted to the Regimen of Health.[1] As such, it is of value, especially to all connected with St Bartholomew's, for it shows the theory upon which treatment at the Hospital must have been based in medieval days. The general exhortation to physical exercise, moreover, will be found a prescription pleasant and acceptable to the modern mind.

On examining the chapter it will be found to divide itself naturally into two parts, the first dealing with professional etiquette, and the second containing general rules for preserving health. The unusual length of the first part, as compared with the second, would naturally attract attention, and provoke discussion, even if this were not in itself necessary to the elucidation of the chapter.

Many medical writers, such as Hali Abbas, prefixed their works with some general remarks on the attainments and conduct required of medical men. Mirfeld's maxims for the deportment of the physician when in the house of his patient (which can also be found in Mirfeld's contemporary, John of Arderne) are copied almost verbatim from a passage in the *Cyrurgia* of William de Saliceto. This itself seems to be based directly upon the *Visit of the Physician to the Patient* of Archimatthaeus the Salernitan (who lived about A.D. 1100) and can be traced back, through writers such as these, to the "Hippocratic oath" and the school which gave it birth.

[1] See *infra* pp. 113, 135, 145.

Why, however, should Mirfeld expand this section to such a length? The obvious explanation is that since he himself was a priest who lived in a priory of Augustinian Canons—a religious order which particularly concerned itself with the care of the sick poor in order to direct their thoughts to spiritual matters—and that since he probably expected his work to be circulated among the other houses of the Order, he therefore expounded more especially those charitable ideals, with which he had been brought into contact at St Bartholomew's, and which would naturally appeal to his sacerdotal mind.

The method upon which this part of the chapter is compiled, however, envisages the probability that Mirfeld, whilst incorporating his own denunciations of avaricious physicians, has actually based his work upon that of Humbertus de Romanis, fifth Rector-General of the Dominican Order (1254–1263), who compiled a book which was intended as a guide to the speedy composition of sermons. Examples are given by Humbertus of suggested types of sermons to suit a wide range of individuals, one of them being entitled, "To Medical Students". This sermon opens, curiously enough, with the identical words used by Mirfeld as a theme, i.e. "Nota satis et autentica est historia, etc.",[1] and then continues with the quotation from the Apocrypha, and proceeds to treat of the duties of a physician from the point of view both of the body and of the soul, stressing, as Mirfeld does, the precepts of charity and of adherence to the Canon Law. Whilst it cannot be stated definitely that Mirfeld followed Humbertus, it would be quite in accordance with medieval practice in general and with his own methods in particular, that he should base himself upon such an authority.

Even, however, if Mirfeld followed Humbertus in the

[1] *Infra* p. 122.

arrangement of his matter, he has himself added a series of scathing comments on the morality of his contemporaries. This, although not quite unusual in the diatribes of his period, provides an interesting picture not only of the moral atmosphere in which the medical practitioner was theoretically expected to do his work, but also of the actual manner in which he reacted to his surroundings, and as such merits attention.

The dominating factor in the history of medieval Western Europe was the supremacy of the Church in every department of life and over every form of activity, whether spiritual or physical. This supremacy, moreover, could always be effectively maintained by the administration of the Canon Law with its sanctions, including a penalty such as excommunication, which involved those who incurred it not only in spiritual, but also in social and business ostracism. This elaborate moral code had been gradually developed by the faithful labours of a succession of able jurists, who had fused into one mass the published canons of the General Councils of the Church and the no less important decisions of the Popes. Thus, by the end of the fourteenth century the Church possessed a weapon which, whenever it was used honestly, and not in the manner familiar to all readers of the *Canterbury Tales*, was most effective against every form of moral lapse; for the Canon Law bound both clergy and laity alike, and existed side by side with, and was as effective as, the State Law of every Western European land. It was unlikely that the Church would neglect to supervise the activities of those possessed of such potentialities for good or for evil as were the medical practitioners, and consequently the physician became a subject of attention at a comparatively early date.

The early Fathers of the Church seem to have regarded the physician with disfavour, suspecting, perhaps, his

Pagan ancestry; nor were their successors likely to show
any cordiality to a profession which looked for guidance to
the Moslem Arabians, upon whom had fallen the mantle of
the Greek physicians. Perhaps the early Fathers were in-
fluenced by the idea that loss of bodily health was the result of Sin. At any rate, they seem to have exhorted the
Christian who was stricken down with disease to send, not
for the physician, but for the priest, who would teach him
to seek a cure by means of prayer and fasting. This practice
is apparently based upon the text in St James' Epistle,
ch. 5, vv. 14 and 15:

Is any sick among you? let him call for the elders of the
church, and let them pray over him....And the prayer of
faith shall save the sick, and the Lord shall raise him up.

Hence grew up the service of Extreme Unction, or the
anointing of the sick with consecrated oil, which, although
it came to be deferred until death was imminent, was
originally intended for the cure of the body as well as for
the salvation of the soul; a fact which is pointed out in the
chapter in the *Florarium* which deals with Extreme Unction.

So too developed the idea that it was the function of the
priest, rather than of the medical practitioner, to deal with
those classes of disease which were thought to be due to
supernatural agency, e.g. "possession by devils"; and,
partly for this reason, and partly to protect his flock against
the evil influence of sorcerers and magicians, an aspirant
to the higher ranks of the priesthood had first to become an
"Exorcist" and to familiarise himself with the service that
was specially drawn up for his use.

Whatever may have been the theory of the leaders, there
is no doubt, however, that the practice of the rank and file
of the Church was to call in the physician when necessary.
Moreover, it was soon found that the clergy themselves
were acting as physicians, partly out of charity, but chiefly

owing to the fact that, as a general rule, to them alone belonged the education necessary to attain to mastery of the
books in which the healing art was expounded. At that
period indeed it was almost essential for anybody, who
desired to become lettered, to receive what was known as
the "first tonsure", or in other words to enter the lowest
rank of the priestly class.

So long as these men remained in the "minor orders",
i.e. those of "Doorkeeper", "Reader", "Exorcist", and
"Acolyte", their practice of Medicine could cause no grave
concern to their superiors. The position was otherwise,
however, when they desired to enter, or were already
members of the "major" or "holy" orders of the priesthood, to which alone pertained the privilege of assisting in
the administration of the Sacraments of the Church. For it
was obvious to the authorities that an honest but inefficient
physician might easily be responsible for the death of a
patient, or if not for his death, at least for his mutilation
(as the severance or destruction of one of the principal
members was termed). The priest, however, who caused
the death or mutilation of a human being, was considered
to have human blood on his hands and was held to have
"become irregular", or to have "incurred an irregularity",
as it was termed; that is, he became automatically incapable of performing the highest functions of the priestly
office and of administering the Sacraments.

The danger of numerous priest-physicians becoming
irregular, and the inconvenience, if not scandal, which
would result therefrom, led the ecclesiastical authorities to
look with disfavour upon the practice of Medicine or
Surgery by those in "major" orders. The consequence
was a series of enactments (among which may be cited that
of the Council of Rheims in A.D. 1131) which, beginning
by merely preventing priests and monks from attending

public lectures in Medicine and permitting private study, terminated eventually in that canon of the Fourth Lateran Council (A.D. 1215) which ordered all subdeacons, deacons, and priests to abstain from the practice of Surgery, especially that which involved burning or cutting, the penalty for disobedience being excommunication. Pope Honorius III (1216–1227) extended this prohibition to the practice of Medicine.

Such a regulation did not, of course, apply to those who were in the lower orders (although a man whose culpable negligence had caused the death of a patient was held to be an homicide and incapable of proceeding to the higher orders); nor did the Church wish to oppose the practitioners of the Healing Art: on the contrary, no less a person than the famous physician, Petrus Hispanus, the reputed author of the *Thesaurus Pauperum*, became Pope, in 1276, under the title of John XXI: and actually during the opening years of the century in which John Mirfeld lived, a parson, Nicholas Tyngewich,[1] was acting as physician to King Edward I of England. The rise of the Universities, however, led to the growth of a large class of persons who took minor orders as a means of obtaining the social and legal privileges granted to the members of the clerical classes. These men regarded the practice of Medicine, not as the performance of a charitable service, but as the means of obtaining a livelihood, and did not always concern themselves about the souls of their patients.

Moreover, to these was added an ever-increasing number of physicians who were actually laymen, who would neither be expected nor permitted to handle matters spiritual. Consequently the framers of the Canon Law drew up regulations for the conduct of such people, and insisted that they should call in the priest in cases where the patient was in

[1] Mentioned in the *Breviarium* (see p. 21).

danger of death, forbidding them to advise any infraction of the Decalogue, and not permitting the acceptance of fees from the poor. A cleric, indeed, was never allowed to ask for a fee, although he might accept one from a rich patient, provided it were spontaneously offered. In practice, as we find from Mirfeld's diatribes, these regulations were honoured more in the breach than in the observance. The priestly compiler of the *Florarium*, however, writing as he did in an Augustinian cloister, was primarily concerned with maintaining the moral idealism of medical practitioners in an age which was notorious for its laxity, and this is the reason why this aspect of his subject is treated at such length.

Having thus delivered himself of his obligations with respect to the soul, our author then proceeds to the body, and gives general advice on the maintenance of health.

As is only fitting, Mirfeld opens his general remarks on the preservation of health with some quotations from the popular medieval poem on that subject, namely the *School of Salerno*. He then proceeds to quote another well-known treatise of a general nature upon which the *School of Salerno* seems to be based; for it is now recognised that part, at least, of the poem is, in its shorter form, little more than a rhymed version of part of another work which dates back to the seventh or eighth century. This is the Pseudo-Aristotelian *Secretum Secretorum*, or *Secret of Secrets*, which its editor, R. Steele, considers to have been originally written in Syriac, and from thence translated into Arabic. This work purports to be a letter written by Aristotle to Alexander the Great, in which the philosopher proposes to initiate the monarch into those secrets which he has hitherto guarded from the knowledge of the world. It is in effect little more than an encyclopaedia compiled for the guidance of a king or an administrator.[1] Nothing is known of its origin beyond the fact that it is no longer considered to be the work of the man whose name it bears; for the ascription to Aristotle, coloured by insertion in the preface of a fabricated story of the accidental discovery of the book in a temple, was simply a fiction intended to supply the work with the prestige of a great name, the writings of Aristotle being always sure of a hearty welcome from the Arabians.

The *Secretum* exists in several versions, but these all contain a section devoted to the maintenance of health; and this medical portion was partly translated into Latin (from the "Western" version) by Johannes Hispaliensis, a Jewish convert to Christianity who flourished at Toledo somewhere about A.D. 1135–1153. It is upon this translation by John of Toledo, which, like all other versions of the *Secretum*, is in prose, that the versified *School of Salerno* is based, and the two works vied with each other for the popularity of the general public during the Middle Ages. On referring to Mirfeld's works it will be found that he uses both versions impartially. Opening the medical section of his chapter in the *Florarium* with verses from the *School of Salerno*, he proceeds to the quotation of its great prose rival and ancestor; he then returns again to his first choice, and after that treats the two authorities as one work to such an extent that it sometimes becomes difficult to disentangle them.

Having opened his general remarks on the maintenance of health by quoting the two most popular general works of his age, viz. the *Secretum Secretorum* and the *Schola Salernitana*, Mirfeld now proceeds to details, and he therefore, in the typical medieval manner, strings together quotations from the books of those Arabians and others of whom mention has already been made. In this he was fortunate in

[1] It is interesting to note that an illuminated copy of the *Secretum Secretorum*, now in the Library at Holkham, was executed for King Edward III.

having the task already completed for him, and at his hand: for although Sir Norman Moore seems to have considered the remainder of the chapter from the *Florarium* to be an original production, the fact must have escaped his notice that the residue of Mirfeld's work—with the exception of the insertion of part of the text of Isaac Judaeus on *Particular Diets*, and the return to the theological character at the finish—is, in effect, simply a series of disjointed excerpts from one of the minor works of a well-known medical author, Bernardus de Gordonio.

This famous physician became Professor of Medicine in the University of Montpellier in A.D. 1285, and (as has been stated above) in the year 1305 he published his *Lilium Medicine*, which became so justly famous. The favourable reception accorded to the *Lilium* led to the publication, in 1307, of another book which, as Bernardus informs us in the preface, was commenced on the 22nd of February, 1307, and finished on the 9th of November in the same year. This work was the *De Conservatione Vite Humane*, which was formerly regarded as four separate treatises, but has now been shown to be but one book composed in four sections;[1] and it is from the "Second Age" (i.e. Youth) of the "Fourth Particula", or "Regimen Sanitatis" of this compilation that Mirfeld's haphazard extracts are taken. A fuller series of quotations from the same work is also to be met with in the first "Distinction" of Part xv of the *Breviarium*, namely that devoted to the "Regimen of Health".

Finally, as is appropriate, Mirfeld returns again to the Bible.

[1] By H. I. Bell in *Proceedings of the Nineteenth International Congress of Medicine*, 1925.

II. PROEMIUM

FLORARIUM BARTHOLOMEI

Gracias ago gracie Largitori quia gratanter audisti frater karissime ea que edificant ad salutem. Vnde etiam contigit vt curialium sollicitudinum [curiosas occupaciones et periculosas vexationes et mercatorum secularium laboriosa][1] euasisti certamina Vt iam opprimens sarcina deposita liberius in lege domini meditari et quiescius leccioni et scripture sacre et oracioni valeas indulgere. Vnde et optasti vt in breui tibi volumine scriberem normam[2] recte viuendi et diuine legis precepta et eius saluberrima consilia. Sed vt verum fatear hoc quod desideras a me iam tibi fieri valde difficile et inconueniens est mihi, videlicet, vt ego tenebrosum cor gerens et propria malicia excecatum viam veritatis et perfectionis alicui propria ostendam industria; qui quidem quasi continue ab exordio iuuentutis mee per deuia voluptatum et abrupta viciorum in inuio semper et non in via oberrans infinitis me miscui malis. Sed quia totaliter negare non possum quod iniungis caritate Christi compulsus et multiplicibus beneficiis tuis obligatus, tua cupiens implere desideria spem habens tuis oracionibus auxilio fulciri diuino multas et precipuas auctoritates et nobilissimas notabilitates quas vnquam in scripturis sacris et virorum catholicorum opusculis reperi quas apud me in sedulis et membranulis non paucis confuse collectas habui in vna hic summula quasi in quodam repositorio seriatim sub certis curaui distinguere capitulis secundum ordinem elementorum alphabeti prout in fine libri patebit manifeste. Nichil in ea omnino de meo nisi tamen seriem et rubricas apponendo sed quod maiorum commendat tradicio.

Et illas precipue collegi et inserui hic notabilitates que specialius vt mihi videbatur possent lectorem instruere de

[1] *Sic* in MS. A. In B this is "periculosas operaciones et intricatorum secularium negotiorum laboriosa", and in E it is "periculosas occupaciones et intricatorum secularium negotiorum laboriosa".   [2] "formam" in MS. B.

THE PREFACE

FLORARIUM BARTHOLOMEI

I give thanks to the Giver of Grace, O Dearest Brother,[1] that
you have willingly hearkened to those things which edify unto
salvation, from whence it has come about that you have
escaped from the strifes and anxieties of the courtiers, from
occupations productive of care and danger, and from the
wearisome vexations of intricate secular business; and that
now, having made an end of these things, and having cast away
your burden of care, you are able to indulge yourself more
freely in meditation upon the Law of God, as well as in more
peaceable reading of the Holy Scriptures, and in prayer.

You have therefore desired me to set down for you, in one
small book, that which is the pattern of the righteous life, as
well as the precepts and most beneficial counsels of the Divine
Law. I must, however, truly confess that what you have desired
me to do for you is most difficult and unbefitting; namely, that
I, with my heart darkened and blinded by my own wickedness,
should endeavour by my own efforts to point out the way of truth
and perfection to another soul; I, indeed, who, as it were, continuously from my youth up, have strayed always not on the
highway but in the by-way, and wandering along the paths of
desire and through the pit-falls of vice, have mixed myself up
with a multitude of evils. I cannot, however, deny what you
would have of me, since I am compelled both by the love of
Christ and by the numerous obligations which I am under to
you; and thus, desiring to fulfil your wishes, and hoping by
means of your prayers to be supported with Divine assistance,
I have collected together here many of the principal, noteworthy, and most noble precepts, which I have ever found in
the Holy Scriptures or in the works of Catholic writers, and
of which I have had by me a disordered collection on many
loose sheets and little scraps of parchment; and I have taken
care to arrange them here in this one little summary, as in a
kind of repository, in a series of chapters in alphabetical order,
as will be seen at the end of the book.[2] And certainly nothing
in it is my own work, except the serial arrangement and the
titles, for it contains only what the voice of Tradition commends.

Moreover, I have particularly collected and inserted here
those noteworthy sayings which seemed to me to be more
specially useful in instructing the reader concerning the empty

---

[1] I.e. John de Suthwell, see Acrostic, p. 100.   [2] See p. 164.

vana et misera mutabilitate huius seculi, de vera et beata
stabilitate futuri, et etiam vt amatores mundi periclitantes
in eo quasi in speculo hic clare videant qualiter neglecta
vita ad interitum tendant. Vbi iaceant quomodo vel
quando assurgant quid cauere quid ve appetere debeant
Et vt beatitudinem quam inter vana peritura querunt nec
inueniunt in sola bonitate diuina et eternorum bonorum
desiderio inuenire se posse confidant. Et omnia pene que
in hac compendiosa compilacione continentur in scripturis
autenticis credo contineri. Que si placet compilacio integra
vocitetur Florarium Bartholomei. Florarium enim secundum grammaticos dicitur locus vbi flores habundant
Et ego flores quos in campo florigero scripturarum sacrarum et spiritualium elegi doctorum et sapientium virorum
quasi ex agricolarum ortis in vnam preciosam hic collegi
massam vt in vnum congesti locum ad dulcorandum legen-
tium corda quasi rosarum flores suauem reddant odorem.
Sed quare cum hac additione Bartholomei sic nominatur
Ad presens nolo declarare; non expedit quidem.

Porro sine aliquorum vtilitate esse non arbitror tam
preciosa scripturarum verba sacrarum in vno volumine
contineri. Hec est enim diuinorum pigmentorum Apotheca
delectabilis. In hoc etenim volumine potest homo doceri
deum cognoscere diabolo resistere et caritatis exerciciis
insudare.

Opus inquam presens siue intentio compilatoris est omni
instantia persuadere amatores mundi quatinus relictis
immoderatis cupiditatibus suis cum omnibus aliis viciis
per sancte pauperitatis et virtutis[1] vias reuerti studeant
ad gratiam redemptoris quam fugiunt mundi   Et vt paucis
multa concludanda sicut in Apotheca diuitis alicuius omnis
homo quod desiderat inuenit sic et in ista compilacione
omnis anima Christiana quod necessarium habet ad morum
honestatem et anime sue salutem implicite vel explicite
inuenire potest diligens inuestigator. Vtere igitur Amice
karissime presenti opusculo vice speculi in quo feda et

    [1] "salutis" in MS. B.

and wretched mutability of this present life, and the true and blessed stability of the life to come; that those lovers of this world, who are jeopardising their eternal safety, may be able to perceive here clearly, as in a mirror, how, by neglecting the true life they are heading for destruction; where they may fall, when or by what manner they may rise; what they ought to heed, or what they ought to desire, and how they may be assured of finding that blessedness, which they seek amongst vanities which shall perish, in the Divine Excellence alone, and in the desire of those things which are of eternal goodness.

And I believe that almost everything which is contained in this compendious compilation can be found in works of acknowledged authority. And let the whole collection, if it pleases, be called "Florarium Bartholomei", that is "The Flower-garden of Bartholomew". A flower garden, according to the grammarians, is a place where flowers abound. And I have chosen the flowers from the flower-bearing field of sacred writings, and of spiritual teachers, and of wise men, as if from the gardens of cultivators, and have gathered them here in one precious collection, and in one place, to delight the hearts of the readers, just as the flowers of roses do give forth a sweet odour: but wherefore with this addition "Bartholomew" to the title I do not wish to say at present; nor indeed would it be expedient.

Furthermore, I do not consider that such precious words of Holy Scripture contained in one volume can be entirely without use. This is indeed a delightful storehouse of divine adornments, for in this volume a man can be brought to the knowledge of God, taught to resist the devil, and to be untiring in the works of charity. I say that the purpose of the present work and the intention of the compiler is by every means to persuade lovers of this world, that, having left behind them as much as possible their immoderate desires and all other vices, they may, by the paths of holy poverty and virtue, study to return again to the grace of the Redeemer of the world, from which they now flee. And just as, by shutting up many things in a small space, as in the storehouse of a rich man, every one finds whatever he may desire, so in this compilation may the diligent investigator find that which every Christian soul needs for its virtuous behaviour and its salvation, implicitly or explicitly set forth. Therefore, Dearest Friend, make use of this present little work just as you would a mirror ("speculum") in which you may clearly see and feel both the ugliness and the beauty of your mind, and by which you may clearly perceive what progress you are making and how far you have gone along the

pulcra mentis tue clare prospicies sencies que dilucide
quantum proficis quantum ve a profectu longe sis vt feda
quecumque corrigas pulcraque conseruando pulcriora
facias. Et non inmerito vt reor speculo potest comparari
cum feda ostendat et corrigere doceat.

Non te moneat frater karissime compilatoris siue scribentis
autoritas nec quis sit sed quid scripsit intende diligentius
nec super verbis infrascriptis facias questionem de qua
scilicet auctoritate sumantur dummodo veritati diuine legis
conueniant et edificent ad salutem. Nam nec de herba
queritur qua scilicet terra vel cuius ortolani cura et cultura
adolerit dummodo vim habeat sanatiuam. Autoritates
siquidem quantum ad librorum capitula non potui de-
terminate assignare cum in diuersis libris diuersi mode
capitula signentur   Et sepe eadem Autoritas a diuersis
doctoribus scribitur quomodo vna et eadem auctoritas ab
eodem in diuersis locis frequenter inuenitur. Sed omne
verbum doctrine catholice consonum a quocumque dicatur
a spiritu sancto est. Nomina autem Autorum quorum dicta
hic sepius allegantur in libri huius marginibus pro maiore
parte inuenies seriatim nec tediosum obsecro tibi videatur
si vnam et eandem Autoritatem in diuersis hic capitulis
inueneris recitatam cum sepe vna clausula pluribus
conueniat materiis nec dicas propter hoc esse nugacio que
est inutilis repeticio vnius et eiusdem   Quoniam secundum
venerabilem Bedam non ab re est sepius verbum repetere
quod semper est necesse animo retinere   Et vt ait Ouidius
decies repetita placebunt. Legant ergo vt scribitur qui
volunt et qui nolunt omittant. Propter calumpniatores
non dimittam magis enim tuo pio desiderio prouocabor
ad studium quam eorum detractione deterrebor non vero
affectans laudes hominum nec nichilominus vituperaciones
expauescens sed deo placere cupiens minas hominum
aut derisas eorum penitus non timebo Quoniam dis-
sipat deus ossa eorum qui hominibus placere desiderant.

road leading to salvation; so that by correcting what is foul and preserving what is beautiful, you may attain to greater beauty. And indeed I think that this can deservedly be compared to a mirror, since it shows forth the foulness of one who gazes upon it, and teaches how the same may be corrected.

Let not, Dearest Brother, your mind be troubled by any question as to the authority of the compiler or writer nor who he is[1]; but study more attentively what he has written; and do not make any question concerning what is written below (namely, as to the authority from which it is taken) provided that it is in agreement with the Divine Law and profitable unto salvation. For it is not demanded of a herb from what ground or under whose care and cultivation it has grown up, provided that it possesses the required healing virtue. And if, indeed, I was not able to cite accurately the chapter of some of my authorities, since the division into chapters is not always the same in every copy of a work, and often the same authority is cited by different doctors in such a way that one and the same authority is found frequently in many places by the same man; nevertheless, every word that is in conformity with Catholic doctrine, by whomsoever it is spoken, is inspired by the Holy Spirit. For the most part, however, you will find the names of the authors whose words are the more frequently quoted set out in order in the margins of this book, and I pray that it may not prove tiresome to you should you find one and the same Authority cited here in various chapters, since one small clause often applies to many matters; and do not say that this repetition of one and the same thing is worthless and useless. For according to the Venerable Bede it is not useless to repeat something more than once, for this is always necessary for the purpose of retaining it in the mind. And, as Ovid says, "Whatever is ten times repeated shall bring pleasure".

Let those, therefore, who wish to do so, read what is written, and let those who do not, leave it alone. I shall not desist from this task on account of those persons who will abuse me; I shall rather be stimulated to study by your devout wishes than deterred by their evil speaking. For indeed I seek not the praises of men,[2] nor indeed do I heed their abuse; but desiring merely to please God I shall have no fear in my heart of the threats or derision of mankind: for God scattereth the bones of those who

---

[1] "Peter of Blois" in the margin of MSS.
[2] St Jerome, Prologue to the Book of Esther. Printed, Migne, *Patrologia Latina*, xxviii, 1434.

Et secundum Apostolum qui huiusmodi sunt serui Christi
esse non possunt. Verum tamen obsecro vt nulli homini
huius opusculi compilatoris nomen patefacias ne ex in-
sipiencia compilatoris et persone vilitate opusculi huius
labor vilescat intuenti sed et illis ad legendum accomoda
si velis qui volunt animum intendere et discere quemadmodum oporteat mores instituere qui secundum legem
dei proposuerunt vitam agere irreprehensibilem.

Prius tamen rogo te amice karissime per eam caritatem
qua me diligis vt libellum hunc diligenter examines et si
que corrigenda sunt corrigas et que radenda sunt radas et
que melius ordinanda sunt ordinare velis antequam in
manus multorum veniens publicetur. Etiam tunc beatus
plane erit qui in istis versatur bonis que in isto continentur
volumine. Qui vero ponit ea in corde suo sapiens erit
semper ac siquidem hec fecerit ad omnia valebit quia lex
dei nostri eius vestigia illuminabit et ministrabit illi cordis
iocunditatem et pacis tranquillitatem per dies sempiternos.

Intelligite nichilominus quod Autoritates subscripte que
ad excitandam legentis mentem ad amorem dei vel
timorem seu ad suimet discussionem hic vtique compilate
sunt non sunt legende in tumultu sed in quiete nec velociter
sed tractatim cum intenta et morosa meditatione nec debet
intendere lector vt multum legat inde vna vice sed quantum
sentit sibi deo inspirante et adiuuante valere ad accen-
dendam cordis affectionem et mentis deuocionem vel quantum illi delectat spiritualiter ne prolixitas lectionis generet
fastidium sed pocius vt aliquem inde colligat lector pietatis
affectionem et luculente discrecionis intellectum. Manifestato
iam prohemio attendendum est ad librum Et quia inter
subscripta capitula secundum ordinem Alphabeti Abstinencia primum occupat locum insuper et nullus palmam
certaminis spiritualis apprehendet vt ait beatus Gregorius
qui non in semetipso prius per afflictam mentis concupi-
scenciam carnis insentiue deuicerit ideo ad capitulum de
abstinencia conueniencius esse videtur inchoandum.

desire only to please men.[1] And according to the Apostle men
of this nature cannot be the servants of Christ.[2] Notwith-
standing this, however, I beseech you that you make known
the name of the writer of this work to no man, lest by the foolish-
ness of the compiler and the worthlessness of his person, the
labour of this work shall be cheapened in the sight of the be-
holder. To those, however, who are willing to turn their minds
upon it and to learn what is necessary for instruction in morals,
and who propose to live a blameless life; to these, if you wish,
you may lend it to read.

However, I ask of you, my dearest friend, by that love which
you bear towards me, that you will previously examine this my
little book, and whatever you find needing correction, then
amend it; and whatever needs excision, cut it out; and whatever
requires a better arrangement, alter it, before it shall be published
abroad. And he will be indeed blessed who busies himself with
the good things that are contained in this volume. Whosoever
establishes them in his heart will always be possessed of wisdom,
and whoever does this will be able to accomplish all things, for
the law of our God shall be a light unto his path, and shall
bring him joy of heart and calmness of peace for evermore.

Understand, however, that the authorities given below,
since they are compiled for the stimulation of the mind of the
reader to the love and fear of God, and to the consideration of
Him, are not to be read amidst tumults, but in quiet; not
speedily, but one subject at a time, with intent and thoughtful
meditation; nor should the reader attempt more at one sitting
than he feels to be, by the inspiration and help of God, of value
in kindling the affection of his heart and the devotion of his
soul, and in providing him with spiritual enjoyment; lest a
superabundance of reading should generate distaste; but rather
that the reader should gather from it a love of piety and a clear
understanding of discretion.

The Preface having been thus set forth, I must now proceed
to the book itself: and because amongst the underwritten chapters, that on "Abstinence" occupies the first place according
to the alphabetical arrangement; because, moreover, nobody
attains to the palm in the spiritual conflict who does not first, as
the Blessed Gregory says, cleanse away the filthy sins of the
body by first overcoming the abominable desires of the mind;
therefore it would seem most fitting to lay the foundation stone
of the work with the chapter on "Abstinence".

[1] Psalm (Vulgate text) 52, v. 6.   [2] St Paul, Epistle to Galatians, ch. 1, v. 10.

III. Chapter: DE MEDICIS ET EORUM MEDICINIS

FLORARIUM BARTHOLOMEI

(Capit. LXXXVIII)

Nota satis et autentica est historia que ait, Altissimus de terra creauit medicinam et vir prudens non abhorrebit illam. Honora, inquit, medicum, propter necessitatem, etenim illum creauit Altissimus. A deo est enim omnis medela, et a rege accipiet donacionem. Disciplina medici exaltabit capud illius et in conspectu magnatorum collaudabitur. Da locum medico, ait sapiens, etenim illum dominus creauit, et non discedat a te, quia opera eius sunt necessaria. Erit enim tempus quando in manibus eius incurras.

Oportet autem quod bonus medicus habeat in se istas tres condiciones quas ponit Haly, scilicet quod sit sciens et diligens et quod operetur secundum artem. Necesse est enim vt medici sint viri litterati aut quod ab eo qui nouit litteras ad minus artem addiscant; vix enim aliquem absque litteratura officium medicorum debite exercere puto; sed tempore presenti nedum ydiote, verumtamen quod deterius est et horribilius iudicatur, viles femine et presumptuose istud officium sibi vsurpant et abutantur eo, que nec artem nec ingenium habent, vnde propter causam sue stoliditatis errores maximos operantur, quibus egri multociens interficiuntur, cum non sapienter nec sub certa radice sed casualiter operantur, et causas et nomina infirmitatum quas asserunt se sanare scire et posse penitus non agnoscunt.[1]

---

¹ "cognoscunt" in MSS. B and D.

---

¹ Ecclesiasticus (Vulgate Text), c. 38, vv. 1–4, 11–13.
² In fact, however, this passage is not taken directly from the Introduction to the *al-Malikī* or *Royal Book* of Hali Abbas, but is an extract from the opening section of the *De Decem Ingeniis Curandorum Morborum* of Bernardus de Gordonio, itself an abstract of Hali.
³ "Wise" in B. de Gordonio, i.e. able to interpret Hippocrates and Galen.
⁴ I.e. visiting patients regularly.
⁵ I.e. according to the canons of Hippocrates and Galen.
⁶ This paragraph and the doleful lament contained therein is copied word for word from the *Magna Chirurgica* of Bruno of Calabria (*circ.* A.D. 1252). At "sed tempore presenti" occurs the note in the margin of C: "Nota hic contra laycos et feminas qui se intromittunt de Phisica". For an example of a medieval "idiota", who was a contemporary of Mirfeld, see H. T. Riley, *Memorials of London*, p. 464, where there is an amusing account

PHYSICIANS AND THEIR MEDICINES

FLORARIUM BARTHOLOMEI

(Chapter 88)

There is a text, sufficiently well known and authenticated, which says,[1] "The Most High created Medicine out of the earth, and a prudent man will not reject it! Honour the physician!" says he, "for thou hast need of him; for the Most High hath created him. Of God cometh all healing; and from the king he shall receive a gift. The skill of the physician shall lift up his head, and in the sight of great men he shall be praised abundantly. 'Give place to the physician', says the wise man, 'for God hath created him, and let him not depart from thee, for his labours are necessary, and there will come a time when thou must fall into his hands'".

Hali Abbas[2] maintains that a good physician should possess three qualifications, namely, that he should be skilful,[3] and diligent,[4] and that he should work in accordance with the generally accepted rules.[5] [6]It is necessary, moreover, that medical men should be well educated, or at least that they should learn their profession from a man of literary attainments; for I consider that an illiterate person is hardly capable of competently performing the functions of a physician. Nevertheless, at the present time, ignorant amateurs, to say nothing of—what is worse, and is considered by me more horrible—worthless and presumptuous women, usurp this profession to themselves and abuse it; who, possessing neither natural ability nor professional knowledge, make the greatest possible mistakes (thanks to their stupidity) and very often kill their patients; for they work without wisdom and from no certain foundation, but in a casual fashion, nor are they thoroughly acquainted with the causes or even the names of the maladies which they claim that they are competent to cure.[6]

of how Roger Clerk, of Wandsworth, was haled before the City justices on the 13th of May 1382, for fraudulently posing as a physician, and treating Johanna, wife of Roger atte Hacche, for fever, by wrapping up an inscribed parchment in a piece of cloth of gold, and telling her to wear it about her neck. When this document was produced in court, Clerk was asked what it signified. He answered that it was a charm written in Latin, and beginning "Anima Christi, sanctifica me; Corpus Christi, salva me" ("Soul of Christ, O sanctify me!; body of Christ, O save me!"); which was false. Moreover, Roger was proved to be wholly illiterate, and totally ignorant of the Healing Art. Wherefore he was sentenced to ride bareback through the City, to the sound of trumpets, with the parchment and a whetstone about his neck, and the utensils of his reputed profession hung before and behind him.

The women were often disreputable quacks, as we see from John of Arderne, Guido de Cauliaco and other writers.

Operanti autem in facultate ista secundum artem et
scientiam ista sequencia sunt necessaria, videlicet, quod
diligenter consideret et inuestiget vt morbi causam cog-
noscat et naturam. Debet insuper medicus acquiescere
voluntatibus[1] infirmorum ex quibus non prouenit detri-
mentum in suis operacionibus, et blandiciis et verbis de-
lectabilibus et suauibus infirmum confortare, et eidem in
omni casu salutem promittere, etiamsi ipse medicus fuerit
de infirmitate desperatus. Nam ex narracione et conforta-
tione tali adquirit anima infirmi disposiccionem nobilem
cum qua natura vigoratur contra infirmitatem et confortatur. Ita quod ex ipsa tunc natura procedit operacio
que est forcior quam sit operacio medici cum instrumentis
et medicinis suis. Sed amicis infirmi veritatem fateatur.
Et cum eis prout ei videbitur melius expedire taliter[2]
loquatur, ne ex ignorancia bone locucionis scandalum incurrat vel infamiam. Et ne amici infirmi malam de eo
habeant suspicionem, et vt non possit dici quod sit causa
mortis eius si moriatur, sed quod sit causa salutis sue qui
viuet et sanabitur. Neque conueniens est vt medicus ser-
monem occultum habeat cum aliqua muliere de domo,
nisi sermo fuerit pro vtilitate operacionis medici circa infirmum. Neque decet eum inhoneste loqui cum eis, nec
affigere aspectum in ipsas temerarium, et maxime coram
infirmo: nam ex hoc nascitur contemptus operacionis eius,
et fides infirmi per prauam ymaginacionem debilitatur et
minuitur. Et ex hoc operacio virtutis naturalis cum medicina vtili et directa pene destruitur, et conuertitur opus
medici in errorem. Nam virtus est que curat infirmitates;
medicus vero non est, sed minister est virtutis. Non seminet
discordiam inter infirmi familiares, nec tribuat ei consilium
non petitum. Non rixetur cum illis de domo, nec aliqua

---

[1] "voluptatibus" in MSS. B and D.   [2] "totaliter" in MSS. B and D.

[1] The text from this point onwards as far as the quotation from the *School
of Salerno* (footnote 2, p. 126) is copied practically verbatim from the

[1] It necessarily follows that a physician who practises his profession in accordance with generally accepted methods and knowledge should make a most careful examination and investigation, so that he may become thoroughly acquainted with both the cause and the nature of the disease with which he has to deal. He should, moreover, permit his patients to indulge themselves in whatever is pleasing to them (provided that this be not prejudicial to his treatment), and by means of blandishments, and of pleasant and soothing speeches, he should comfort his patient, and on every occasion should promise him restoration to health, even if the physician himself shall regard the case as desperate; for by means of such heartening words the sick man is imbued with a courage which strengthens his constitution and fortifies it to resist the disease; so that from Nature[2] herself there proceeds a reaction which is more efficacious than that produced by the physician with his instruments and medicines. Let the physician, however, acquaint the friends of his patient with the truth, and discuss the case fully with them as he shall deem best, lest he incur scandal or loss of reputation from inability to proffer a satisfactory statement of the case, and lest the friends of the patient regard him with distrust: nor will he then be held responsible for having caused the death of a patient who shall die; but he will be given credit for having cured the man who lives and is restored to health.

It is not seemly for the physician to converse in secret with any woman of the patient's household (except it be in connection with his treatment), nor is it consistent with his professional dignity that he should speak shamefully to them or turn bold glances upon them, and particularly when in the presence of the patient. For from this is born contempt for his labours, and the faith of the patient in him is weakened and lessened by his distorted imagination; and in consequence the benefit arising from the skilful use of medicine acting upon the natural tendency to recovery is almost destroyed, and the labour of the physician is turned to reproof. For it is the natural constitution which conquers disease, and not the physician, who is in truth nought but its servant. Let not the physician sow discord among the servants of his patient, nor proffer to the latter unsought advice. Let him not brawl with anybody within the

Introduction to the *Cyrurgia* of William de Saliceto, Professor at Bologna (*flor. circ.* A.D. 1275), which itself is partly an abstract of, and partly a direct quotation from, the *Visit of the Physician to the Patient* of Archimatthaeus the Salernitan (*flor.* A.D. 1100); and is probably based on the Hippocratic corpus.
[2] The "Vis Medicatrix Naturae".

committat inhonesta, vel que hominibus rationabiliter dis-
plicere possunt. Nam omnia hec corrumpunt bonam
opinionem et medicum vilipendunt. Non delectetur in
familiaritate laicorum, laici enim semper medicis detrahere
consueuerunt. Nimia enim familiaritas parit contemptum,
et eciam per nimiam familiaritatem Non sic audacter et
secure petitur remuneracio operacionis. Et scias quod
bona remuneracio de labore et salarium bonum arti-
ficem reddit auctorizabilem et confortatur inde fides infirmi super eum, eciam si multe fuerit ignorancie; ita
quod infirmus opinatur ex hoc quod melius possit aliis et
debeat procedere in cura sua: ideo veredicus versificatur
ait sic:

> Empta solet care multum medicina iuuare.
> Si detur gratis nichil affert vtilitatis.

Pauperes tamen pro posse visitet prout decet.

Medicus autem ad infirmos vocatus pro cura adhibenda
debet ante omnia eos monere et inducere vt aduocent ab
inicio medicos animarum, id est, confessores, vt postquam
fuerit eis de spirituali salute prouisum ad corporalis medicine remedium licite procedatur. Et si quis medicorum
huius statuti fuerit transgressor ab ingressu ecclesie sus-
pendatur donec super transgressione satisfecerit competenter. Nam et hominem dominus a paralisi curaturus
primo peccatorum vincula dissoluit dicens, Homo, re-
mittuntur tibi peccata tua, Vt ostenderet eum ob nexus
culparum artuum dissolucione dampnari, nec nisi hiis re-
laxatis membrorum posse recuperacione sanari. Sic et illi
paralitico qui iuxta probaticam piscinam diu motum aque
frustra prestolabatur, et sanato a domino dicitur, Ecce
sanus factus es: iam noli peccare ne deterius tibi aliquid

---

¹ An old Latin proverb which may be traced to Publilius Syrus (c. B.C. 40).
² MSS. note "versus", i.e. indicating a quotation from the *School of
Salerno* (in the Villanova version) the unknown composer of which is hence-
forward referred to as "The versifier".

house or belonging to the household, nor behave dishonourably
or in a manner which may reasonably give offence. For all
these things destroy the good reputation of the physician, and
cause him to be lightly esteemed.

Let him not take delight in the friendship of laymen, for they
make it their practice to disparage the members of his profession; and further

Too much familiarity doth breed contempt.[1]

Nor can he boldly and securely seek remuneration for his
services from those with whom he has been too intimate.
Moreover, it should be known that a good recompense for his
labour, and a high salary, if demanded, imparts to the physician
an air of authority, which strengthens the confidence of the
patient in him (even though he be particularly ignorant), so
that the sick man imagines from this that he is more skilful
than others and ought therefore to be successful in curing him.[2]
Truly speaks the versifier thereon,

When Physick's dearly bought, it doth much healing bring,
But when 'tis freely given, 'tis ne'er a useful thing.[3]

Let him with diligence attend the poor, however, as is fitting.

[4]The physician, when called in to attend the sick, ought, before everything else, to warn them, and to persuade them at the
outset to call in physicians of the soul, that is to say, Confessors;
and then, when provision has been made for their spiritual
health, he may lawfully proceed to apply his remedy to the
body and make use of medicine. And if any physician shall
disobey this ordinance, let him be forbidden to enter a church
until he has made due amends for his fault. [5]For the Lord,
when about to cure the man sick of the palsy, first loosed from
off him the bonds of his sins, saying unto him,

Man, thy sins are forgiven thee,[6]

in order that He might show him that it was due to the fetters
of his iniquities that he was condemned to weakness of the
joints, and that unless these were first unbound, he could not be
made whole by the recovery of the use of his limbs. So also,
that impotent man who by the side of the sheep-pool had long

[3] *School of Salerno*: De Renzi, ll. 2078, 2079.
[4] Here begin the extracts from the Canon Law: the reference is to the
section "De Poenitentia et Remissione", capit. "Cum infirmitas".
[5] This next section, as far as note 2, p. 128, is copied from the Commentary
of the Venerable Bede on Luke, ch. 2. (In the MSS. it is ascribed to Bede
"in quadam omelia".)
[6] Vulgate, Luke v. 20.

contingat. Et ideo consulte a salamone dicitur Qui dere-
liquit[1] in conspectu eius qui fecit illum incidet in manus
medici. Prohibitum est etiam sub interminacione ana-
thematis ne aliquis medicorum pro corporali[2] salute aliquid
egroto suadeat quod in periculum anime conuertatur. Et
caueat sibi medicus quia si per necgligenciam ipsius mors
euenerit infirmo siue membri mutilacio, irregularis effi-
citur. Et in Canone dicitur quod clericus in sacris ordinibus
constitutus exercens officium cyrurgie excommunicandus
est: non licet ergo clericis in sacris ordinibus constitutis
exercere officium cyrurgie quia non est officium clericale.
Vnde et deponendi[3] sunt.

Medicus autem in medicinis conferendis,[4] sic procedere
debet vt illas exhibeat medicinas quas scit secundum artem
proficere debere   Ita quod omnia diligenter inspiciat consideranda. Peccat enim dando medicinam si dubitat eam
nocituram vel profituram.[5] Similiter ita peccat medicus
omittendo medicinas debitas sicut exhibendo indebitas.
Et si medicus dicat se peritum ad medicandum aliquam
infirmitatem cum non scit, et faciat vel omittat quicquam,
et ob hoc aliquod periculum incurrat infirmus, grauiter
peccat, et fit irregularis in casibus suis: Si autem medicus
certus est quod secundum artem vtile esse aliquem incidi,
secure autem tunc faciat eum incidi dummodo peritum et
discretum inueniat incisorem; nec fit in hoc casu irregularis
quamuis mors inde sequatur, quia forte infirmus non

[1] Sic for "delinquit".   [2] "temporali corporali" in MS. B.
[3] "disponendi" in B.   [4] "confouendis" in B and D.
[5] "Si dubitet esse noscituram vel profuturam" in B.

[1] Vulgate, John, ch. 5, v. 14.
[2] Vulgate, Ecclesiasticus, ch. 38, v. 15.
[3] Canon Law, "Cum infirmitas". This refers to incantations of a pagan
origin, witchcraft, etc., rather than to self-indulgence, although breaches of
the rules relating to fasting were naturally frowned upon.
[4] Canon Law: Decretals of Gratian, section "De Homicidia", capit.
"Tua nos", and section in gloss thereon "Ex hac de causa".
[5] I.e. the Canon of the Lateran Council (1215) (supra p. 110).

awaited in vain the troubling of the water, was thus addressed after he had been healed by the Lord,

Behold,[1] thou art made whole: sin no more lest a worse thing come unto thee.

Therefore it is deliberately said by Solomon,

He who sinneth in the sight of his Maker, shall fall into the hand of the physician.[2]

It is prohibited, under threat of anathema,[3] that any physician should persuade a sick man to do anything for the benefit of his earthly body, which may jeopardise the safety of his eternal soul. And let the physician be on his guard, for he "incurs an irregularity", if by his negligence, the sick man dies, or suffers the mutilation of a limb.[4] And in one of the Canons[5] it is laid down that a "clerk" in Holy Orders who acts as a surgeon, is to be excommunicated;[6] the reason for this being that the performance of the duties of a surgeon is not a clerical function. Wherefore they are to be deprived of office.[7]

The physician, when prescribing, should diligently weigh in his mind everything which demands consideration, so that he may make use only of those remedies which, according to his knowledge, he is confident will produce advantageous results; for he does amiss in prescribing a medicine of which he is in doubt as to whether it will be dangerous or beneficial. Similarly he does wrong in failing to give a medicine that is needful, as well as in giving one that is not required. And if any physician says that he is competent to treat a disease when he is not; and if he does, or does not do, something by reason of which the sick incur danger: then he sins grievously, and is "made irregular" by any consequent disaster.[8] If, however, the physician is convinced that, according to the principles of his Art, a surgical operation would be beneficial, then he may safely order it to be performed, provided that he obtains a skilful and discerning surgeon for his patient; nor does he incur

[6] MSS. note "in Innocent's gloss on this chapter", i.e. the critical apparatus on the five books of the *Decretals* propounded by Pope Innocent IV.

[7] The only possible translation in this context: actually, in the Canon Law, the meaning is "they are to be deposed from their situations" and refers rather to abbots and others in authority who permit those subordinated to them to commit irregularities; it can also refer to the deprivation of beneficed clergy, e.g. on xv Kalends of January 1399, the Pope ordered that Denis Cachaerna, an Irish parish priest having the cure of souls, should be deprived of his canonry and prebend, because he "publicly practises the art of medicine *for money* [our italics] to the opprobrium of his clerical estate" (*Calendar of Entries in the Papal Registers relating to Great Britain and Ireland—Papal Letters*, Vol. v (1396–1404), p. 315).

[8] Canon Law. "Ne clerici vel monachi", cc. i, ii and iii: also "Tua nos", and in Innocent.

habeat consuetam disposicionem membrorum vel venarum. Incisor tamen potius dimittat quam incidat, si in
aliquo dubitet. Securius est enim hominem relinquere in
manibus creatoris sui quam incisioni vel medicine de qua
dubitat quocumque modo. Et scire debes quod medicus
licite promoueri potest, si eum non remordet conscientia.
Ast si conscientia medici ipsum remordet quia forte inperite
medicinam dederat infirmis propter quod mors fuerat
secuta; vel si necgligens fuerit in cura sua, quia dissoluta
necgligencia prope dolum est: Non debet ascendere ad
maiores ordines. Alias euentus mortalis non debet medico
imputari. Caue tibi a medico, ait beatus Bernardus,
volente in te experiri qualiter alios de simili morbo curabit.
Et Seneca, Medicorum, inquit, consilia deuita, qui parum
docti et satis seduli officiosissime multos occidunt. Com-
mune quidem medicorum vicium est semper circa egritu-
dines variare Vnde si tres aut quatuor ad infirmum veniunt
nunquam in assignacione cause vel exhibicione cure conueniunt. Nichil vero curant de infirmo nisi vt pecuniam
congregent et multiplicent. Refertur autem de quodam
medico cui debebantur xiii libre ad tres annos soluende,
Qui cum laboraret in extremis et admoneretur vt con-
fiteretur et eukaristiam sumeret, nichil aliud poterant ab
eo extrahere nisi xiii libras et tres annos.[1] Tres quidem

    [1] Sic in A, C, E. D has "xiij li iij annos". "xiij libri in tribus annis" in B.

---

    [1] Section "De Aetate et Qualitate" (of candidates for Holy Orders):
Innocent on Homicide at "Tua nos".
    [2] "Dolus" is used here in its technical Roman Law sense of the highest
degree of liability possible.
    [3] Not St Bernard of Clairvaux, but Bernard Sylvester (of Chartres,
A.D. 1080(?)–1167), in his Epistle to Raymund, "Super gubernatione rei
familiaris", al. "De Regimine domus familiaeque" (on the management of
the household).
    [4] MSS. note: "Seneca in quadam epistola". This passage has not been
traced in the extant epistles of Seneca, but Sidonius Apollinaris in his Epistle
to his brother-in-law Agricola ([A.D. 461–467], Bk. II, No. XII, Migne, Patr.
Lat. LVIII, 443) has the following passage: "Vitanda sunt etiam plerumque
consilia medicorum assidentium qui parum docti et satis seduli languidos
multos officiosissime occidunt". A consideration of this sentence, taken in

an irregularity even if death should supervene owing, perchance, to the fact that the patient has not the normal arrangement of limbs or of veins. The surgeon, however, should leave the sick man alone rather than operate, if he is in any doubt: for it is safer to leave a man in the hands of his Creator, than to put trust in surgery or medicine concerning which there is any manner of doubt.

And it should be known that a physician may lawfully proceed to "Holy Orders", provided that his conscience does not reproach him for anything:[1] if, however, his conscience pricks him because by chance he has unskilfully prescribed for a patient, so that death has resulted; or if he shall have been negligent in his treatment, since carelessness and negligence in such cases approximate to criminal culpability,[2] he ought not to advance to the higher orders of the priesthood. Otherwise, the death of a patient should not be laid to the charge of his physician.

"Beware of the physician", says the Blessed Bernard,[3] "who wishes to experiment upon thyself how he may cure others suffering from a similar disease." And Seneca[4] speaks thus of physicians,

Shun the counsel of those of them who, being little learned, but zealous enough, most dutifully slay many.

The common fault[5] of physicians is, that when three or four of them come to visit a sick man, they never agree either in defining the cause of the disease, or in the suggested line of treatment. In truth they trouble themselves in no wise about the patient, except it be to collect and pile up fees from him.

There is a story[6] that is told about a certain physician to whom thirteen pounds had been owing for three years; who, when he was at the point of death, and was admonished that he should confess his sins and partake of the Eucharist, could be brought to answer nothing else except "Thirteen pounds" and "Three years".

conjunction with what has preceded it, leads to the conclusion that it is quite possible that Mirfeld, when he wrote, had before him a somewhat illegible manuscript of the *Speculum Naturale* of Vincent of Beauvais (Lib. xxxi, cap. xcix, "Qualiter consilio medici sit vtendum") and that he misread the reference which will be found there. Mirfeld is generally exact in his quotations from Seneca.

[5] This sentence is taken from the letter of Peter of Blois to his friend Peter, a physician.

[6] This tale is at least a century older than Mirfeld, for it appears in two thirteenth-century manuscript collections of stories intended for the embellishment of sermons, viz. Harley MS. 3244, f. 72 b, and Additional MS. 27909 B, f. 4 b, both of which are in the British Museum. Its source has not been traced.

speciales proprietates moderni medici habere dinoscuntur, videlicet, subtiliter mentiri, honeste procedere, et audacter interficere. Medicus vtique si bonus sit christianus, quod raro accidit, non enim in operibus suis ostendunt se esse discipulos Christi, sed Auicenne et Galieni, deberet curare infirmum christianum etiam gratis si infirmus pauper sit, quia plus debet valere apud eum vita illius quam eius pecunia. Et si infirmus dives est, et nichil vult dare adhuc medicus tenetur ipsum curare propriis expensis. Et si conualuerit, repetat expensas suas, quia utiliter gessit negocium eius. Et etiamsi moriatur eger, potest nichilominus debitas expetere expensas, quia sufficit si vtiliter cepit gerere, licet prosper euentus non sit secutus: nec potest ei obici quod causa pietatis fecerit sumptus illos, nisi esset propinquus infirmo. Mortem enim languentibus probatur inferre qui hanc scilicet mortem cum possit non excludit. O miser medice, ait Lanfrancus, qui pro pecunia quam non speras adquirere deseris corpus humanum in mortis laborans periculo, et eum quem secundum legem dei pre omnibus creaturis que sub celo sunt amare et preponderare deberes, Auaricia excecatus de vita vel membris periclitari permittis, cum scis et possis congruum adhibere remedium. Testor dominum, ait ipse de Gordonio, quod nunquam vidi hominem maliciosum in medicina et dolosum operarium qui dimediaret dies suos, nec habet euentum sordida preda bonum.

Videntur[1] vtique medici spirituales moderni deteriores

---

[1] *Sic* in MSS. A, C, D, E, F. "dicuntur" in B.

[1] These men are obviously quoted as being the two leading heathen physicians. The attack upon their humanity does not, however, seem justified by any valid evidence. Compare Chaucer's "Doctor of Physick" who had "little of the Bible", but who "loved gold in especial". A good fee was also much beloved by Mirfeld's contemporary, John of Arderne, who was established in London by 1372.

[2] *Decretals*, LXXX, and gloss thereon.

[3] "O miser medice, ait Lanfrancus." This is apparently a misquotation and a rather misleading interpretation of the passage in the *Cirurgia Magna* of Lanfranc of Milan (the founder of French surgery, and a pupil of William

Modern physicians appear to possess three special qualifications, namely, to be able to lie in a subtle manner, to show an outward honesty, and to kill with audacity. But the physician, if he should happen to be a good Christian (which rarely chances, for by their works they show themselves to be disciples, not of Christ, but of Avicenna and of Galen),[1] ought to cure a Christian patient without making even the slightest charge if the man is poor; for the life of such a man ought to be of more value to the physician than his money.[2] And even if the sick man is wealthy and as yet unwilling to give anything, the physician is nevertheless obliged to cure him at his own expense and then, should the man recover, let him demand his fee again, because he has successfully performed his task; and even if the sick man shall die, he may nevertheless sue for what is due to him, for it is sufficient if he laboured competently, although the result be unfortunate; nor can his claim for payment be barred on the ground that he attended the rich man from motives of charity, unless he should happen to be a relative of his patient. For he who fails to preserve the sick from death,[2] when he is able to do so, is held to have caused their death.

"O wretched physician," says Lanfranc,[3] "who, when thou hast no hope of acquiring money, desertest a human being labouring in peril of death; and one, whom, according to the law of God, thou shouldest love and esteem above all the creatures that are under the heavens, thou permittest, blinded as thou art by thine avarice, to be imperilled in life or limb, when thou hast the knowledge and ability to provide a suitable remedy."

"I call the Lord to witness", says Bernard Gordon[4] himself, "that I have never seen a man, who, being full of wickedness in his medical practice, and crafty in his dealings, lived out half his days, or had the enjoyment of his sordid spoils."

Modern *Spiritual Physicians*[5] seem, it is true, to be even worse

de Saliceto), Doct. III, tract iii, chapter 7, where (in expounding hernia) Lanfranc reprimands unskilful surgeons who, in order to obtain fees, risk their patients' lives by insisting upon operations in cases where competent men would advise against the use of the knife.

[4] In the introduction to the *De Decem Ingeniis Curandorum Morborum*.

[5] At this point in the margin of MS. F occurs the note "contra curatos" showing conclusively that by "spiritual physicians" is meant the ordinary parish priest having the cure of souls, who is naturally expected to visit the sick members of his flock gratis. "Spiritual healing" means not only the casting out of devils, etc. (see Introduction, p. 108), and generally speaking, the work performed by the modern psychologist, but also an elaborate system of prayer, anointing, and administration of the Sacraments, in which the cure of the sick was sought from God; and which, apart from its spiritual aspect, must have been of great value as a means of keeping the thoughts of the patient fixed on the probability of recovery. Such complaints against spiritual physicians are quite common at this (the Wycliffite) period.

etiam corporalibus medicis tribus de causis. Primo, quia
nullorum egrotorum recusant curam quamuis incurabiles
videantur. Secundo, quia licet de arte spiritualis medicine
parum vel nichil nouerint, Curam tamen multorum audacter et presumptuose suscipiunt.[1] Tertio, quia mercedem
ab infirmis auide accipiunt et de infirmis se non intromittunt: hec enim tria in medicis corporum quantum-
cumque mali sint, non solent simul omnia inueniri. Giezi
reprobatur[2] quia gratiam sanitatis Naaman Syro vendidit.
Numquid igitur licitum est medico recipere pecuniam pro
conferenda sanitate? Certum est quod sic, Quia illud
potius dicitur honor quam pretium. Nec recipit pecuniam
pro sanitate danda, cum illud sit gratia, sed pro labore suo;
sicut Magister non recipit pecuniam pro scientia quam dat
sed pro labore suo vel honore suo, non pro premio gratie.
Et licet scriptura dicat, Qui precepta medici contempnit de
vita periclitatur, non tamen omnes volunt nec semper forte
expedit eorum sequi consilium. Istorum tamen versuum
sententiam non contempnas:

> Si tibi deficiant medici, medici tibi fiant
> Hec tria, mens leta, labor,[3] et moderata dieta.

Et iterum versificator sic dicit:

> Si vis incolumen, si vis te reddere sanum,
> Curas tolle graues, irasci crede prophanum.
> Parce mero, cenato parum, nec sit tibi vanum
> Pergere[4] post epulas; sompnum fuge meridianum.
> Non teneas mictum, non cogas fortiter anum.

[1] "accipiunt" in MS. B.   [2] "approbatur" in B.
[3] *Sic* in MSS. The authentic text is "quies" or "requies".
[4] *Sic* in MSS. An obvious mistake: the correct text is "Surgere".

---

[1] Vulgate, IV Kings, ch. 5, v. 26.
[2] From the gloss on the *Decretals*. This is the usual medieval theory as developed by St Thomas Aquinas and others. A man was entitled to receive
remuneration for his labour, according to his station in life, but not for the
superiority of his intelligence over that of his fellow-men, for this was held
to be a gift from God, and therefore not to be bartered for money. Thus the
physician can take a fee for his attendance upon a patient, but must not take
upon himself the credit or recompense for a cure, which is due to God alone.
This theory seems partly based on the story of Simon Magus (Acts, ch. 8)
and partly on Ecclesiasticus, ch. 38, v. 14, where the physician prays God to
prosper the remedies which he gives.

than physicians of the body, and for three reasons. Firstly, because they never decline to undertake a case, although they perceive that it is hopeless. Secondly, because although they know little or nothing of the science of spiritual healing, yet they nevertheless boldly and presumptuously take upon themselves the cure of many patients. Thirdly, because they greedily accept rewards from the sick, nor do they concern themselves about the welfare of their patients. These three particular faults, however, are not usually found all together in Physicians of the Body, however bad they be. Gehazi[1] was reproached because he sold the gift of health to Naaman the Syrian. [2] Is, therefore, the physician never permitted to receive money for conferring health? So it is established; because this is said to be a source of honour rather than of riches. Nor does he receive money for giving health (for that is due to the grace of God) but for his labours; just like a "master" he does not receive money for the knowledge which he gives,[3] but for his exertions, or as a mark of honour, and not as the reward for what is bestowed by the grace of God. And although according to the Scriptures,

He who despises the precepts of the physician, goes in peril of his life,

yet all men are not willing, nor is it always profitable, to follow his advice.[4] Let not such, however, despise the teaching contained in these following verses:

[5] If physicians thou dost lack, let these three doctors be,
Toil,[6] a sparing diet, and mind from care set free.

And again the versifier thus speaks:

[7] If thou wilt safe, and thou wilt healthy be,
Shun heavy care, and wrath, as things unfit for thee.
Drink not neat wine; dine light, nor think it vain
After thy meals to rise;[8] and midday sleep disdain.
But, whate'er thou dost, heed well this golden rule:
Hold not thy water long; strain not thyself at stool.

---

[3] Medieval education was theoretically free.
[4] From this point onwards most of the chapter will be found in the *Breviarium*, Part xv, Dist. 1, "De Regimine Sanitatis" (as a fuller excerpt from Bernardus de Gordonio, *De Conservatione Vite Humane*) where, however, the lines from the *School of Salerno* are postponed until immediately before the extract from the *Secret of Secrets* (note 2, p. 137).
[5] *School of Salerno*, ll. 8, 9.
[6] "Rest", not "toil", is the normal text, but all the MSS. of the *Florarium* and *Breviarium* (Part xv) agree in the reading here given.
[7] *School of Salerno*, ll. 2–6.
[8] The MSS. of both *Florarium* and *Breviarium* have the ridiculous reading "Purgere" (purge) instead of the correct text "Surgere".

Et iterum alibi dicit versificator:

> Temporibus veris modice prandere iuberis,
> Et calor estatis dapibus nocet immoderatis.
> De mensa sume quantum vis tempore brume,
> Autumpni fructus caueas ne sint tibi luctus.

Dicunt enim naturales quod nisi homo sciat artem sanatiuam vt se regat prudenter ac naturaliter non potest venire ad terminum naturalem mortis; immo morietur ante tempus suum naturale. Et ideo dicit Galienus medicorum princeps, Mirabilis est, inquit, scientia sanatiua, que facit hominem viuere senem et sine egritudine vsque ad vltimum senectutis. Ideo Aristotiles in quodam tractatu de regimine sanitatis, scribens Alexandro Magno, ait inter cetera, O Alexander, cum sit hoc corpus corruptibile, visum est michi tibi scribere quedam vtilia ex secretis artis medicine; si ergo hoc exemplar prospexeris et iuxta hunc preciosum ordinem conuersatus fueris, medico non indigebis, exceptis accidentibus bellicis, scilicet, percussionibus et ceteris huiusmodi que omnino vitari non possunt. Oportet ergo te cum a sompno surrexeris, modicum ambulare et membra tua modicum et equaliter extendere, et capud tuum pectere, quia extencio roborat corpus, et pectinacio extrahit vapores ad capud ascendentes a stomacho tempore dormicionis. Deinde laua manus tuas in estate cum aqua frigida, quia hoc restringit et retinet vapores corporis.[1] Et hoc erit quasi excitacio voluntatis ad comedendum. Deinde lauda et adora dominum deum tuum secundum doctrinam legis tue. Cumque voluntas comedendi iuxta horam consuetudinis affuerit, vtere moderato corporis labore, scilicet, deambulando vel equitando per loca alta munda et a lacubus distancia. Tempus autem exercicii corporalis est cum cibus sumptus optime in stomacho venisque digeritur et natura alium cibum appetere incipiat. Tunc enim exercicium tale vel consimile bonum est et vtile. Frangit namque ventositatem, et corroborat corpus atque alleuiat, et calorem stomachi accendit, et constringit compages atque liquefacit residuos et super-

---

[1] *Sic* in MSS. of *Florarium* and *Breviarium*. An obvious mistake for the authentic text "calorem corporis et capitis euaporantem" of the *Secretum Secretorum*.

And again, the rhymer says elsewhere:

[1]In Spring-time thou thy food shalt moderately take,
And Summer's heat will harm thee should thou then rich banquets
    make.
In Winter thou canst eat whate'er delighteth thee,
In Autumn heed thou fruit, lest to thy grief it be.

Natural philosophers say that unless a man is acquainted
with the healing art, so that he may regulate himself prudently
and naturally, he cannot survive until the natural time for his
death, and will certainly die before the allotted span. And
thus speaks Galen, the "Prince of Physicians",

"Wonderful is this healing science", says he, "which enables a man
to live to old age, and, moreover, free from disease to the end of a long
life."

And thus says Aristotle, amongst other things, in a certain
treatise on the "Regimen of Health" addressed to Alexander
the Great:[2]

O Alexander, since this body is corruptible, it has seemed good to
me to write unto thee those things which are useful out of the secrets
of the art of medicine. If, therefore, thou shalt gaze attentively upon
this model, and shalt follow this precious guide, thou shalt not stand
in need of the physician, except for the accidents of war, such as blows,
and other incidents of that nature, which can never be entirely avoided.
It behoves thee, therefore, when thou arisest from sleep, to walk a
little, and moderately and equally to stretch thy limbs, and to comb
thy hair; for the stretching strengthens the body, and the combing
draws forth the vapours which ascended to the head from the
stomach during sleep. Then wash thy hands in cold water during
summer, for this confines and retains the heat of the body and of the
head, which is evaporating away, and will rouse the appetite to
activity. Then praise and worship the Lord thy God according to the
doctrine of thy law. And when the desire for food shall come unto
thee at the accustomed hour, take a moderate amount of bodily
exercise, such as walking or riding through the uplands where the air
is pure and which are also at a distance from stagnant water.[3] The
best time for bodily exercise, however, is when the food which has
been previously taken has been properly digested in the stomach and
the veins,[4] and the appetite has become quickened with desire for
other food; then such or similar exercise is good and useful, for it
disperses flatulence, strengthens and tones up the body, arouses the
heat of the stomach, braces the frame, and liquefies residual and

---

[1] *Regimen Sanitatis Salerni*, ll. 54–57.
[2] I.e. the extract from the Pseudo-Aristotelian *Secret of Secrets* as translated
into Latin by John of Toledo (see p. 111).
[3] Thus avoiding malaria.
[4] I.e. when all the "three digestions" of medieval medicine have been
fully completed (pp. 31, 32).

fluos humores, et tunc descendet cibus super stomachum accensum.

Fulgentius enim discribit exercicium laboris corporalis per modum decoratissimum, dicens, Exercicium est humane vite conseruacio, caloris naturalis lima et excitacio, nature dormientis stimulacio, superfluorum consumpcio, membrorum consolidacio, mors morborum, fuga viciorum, medicina languorum, temporis lucrum, juuentutis debitum, senectutis gaudium, salutis adiutorium, ocii inimicum, et omnium malorum destrictiuum. Ille ergo solus ab exercicio se subtrahat qui felicitatis gaudio vult carere. Auicenna quidem de corporali exercicio scribebat hoc modo. Exercicium, inquit, motus est voluntarius propter quem anelitus fit magnus frequens et voluntarius.[1] Et ideo oportet quod totus sit liber, et operetur secundum suam voluntatem, ideoque carpentariorum agricolarum mercatorum et labor huiusmodi aliorum non est exercicium, quia proprie non est motus voluntarius sed quodammodo coactus. Preterea, burgenses et claustrales ac tales hiis consimiles bene ambulant et diu, sed non est proprie exercicium, quia hanelitus non mutatur. Exercicium autem quippe non dicitur nisi aliquis ex voluntate propria tantum ambulet et ita velociter quod incipiat fatigari, et hanelitus mutari,[2] et tunc statim debet sedere et quiescere, quoniam si vlterius moueretur, non esset nisi pena et fatigacio. Et tale predictum exercicium appellatur temperatum, et accrescunt multa bona corpori propter tale exercicium. Excitatur enim ex hoc calor naturalis, et vigoratur atque augmentatur, et per consequens, appetitiua digestiua atque virtus expulsiua totius corporis roborantur et meliorantur.

Notandum est ergo quod moderatum exercicium corpora moderate calefacit et desiccat. Si autem immoderatum

---

[1] Not in MSS. A or E. *Sic* in B, D and F, a mistake for "necessarius".
The *Breviarium* has the correct reading.
[2] *Sic* in MSS. for "immutari".

superfluous humours so that the food will descend upon a stomach kindled to receive it.

Fulgentius[1] describes the exercise of bodily labour in a most eloquent manner, saying,

Exercise is the preserver of human life, the refiner and arouser of the natural heat, the stimulant to indolent nature, the consumer of superfluities, the bringer of firmness to the limbs, the vanquisher of disease, the banisher of vice, the medicine for weakness, a profitable pastime, the duty of youth, the joy of old age, an aid to health, an enemy to idleness and the dissolver of all ills. Therefore, let him alone discard exercise who wishes to be without the joy of happiness.

Avicenna,[2] indeed, wrote in this manner concerning bodily exercise:

"Exercise", says he, "is voluntary movement by means of which the respiration is necessarily deepened and accelerated."

Thus everything must be done voluntarily, and therefore the labour of carpenters, farmers, merchants, and the like, is not in the strict sense exercise, because it is not performed with a free will, but is to a certain extent enforced. Moreover, burgesses, monks, and such manner of men walk well and for long periods, yet do not strictly speaking take exercise because they do not become short of breath. Exercise, however, cannot correctly be described as such, unless a man walks of his own free will, and that too so swiftly that he begins to feel tired and out of breath; he ought then immediately to sit down and rest, for, if he should continue to move about, this will produce only pain and fatigue. And such exercise as this is called temperate, and is very beneficial to the body; for by its means the natural heat is aroused, strengthened, and increased; and consequently the appetite, and the digestive and expulsive virtues of the whole body are strengthened and improved.

It[3] is to be noted, therefore, that moderate exercise moderately warms and dries up the body, but if, however, it be im-

---

[1] Note in *Florarium* MSS. [St] "Fulgentius in quadam sermone contra otiosos". This extract sometimes appears as a note appended to the text of the *Secret of Secrets* at this point. It occurs here, however, in its proper place as the opening words of ch. VII ("De Exercicio") of the Fourth Particula or *Regimen Sanitatis* of the *De Conservatione Vite Humane* of Bernardus de Gordonio, disjointed excerpts from which now follow continuously. (Ch. VII begins the section of the *Regimen* on the "Second Age", i.e. "Early Manhood"). In the *Breviarium* this extract is postponed until the end of § 2, p. 141.

[2] *Canon*, I, iii, Doct. 2, c. I.

[3] The following sentence is apparently not taken from this identical part of Bernardus de Gordonio: the quotation is resumed at l. 4, p. 141 "but nevertheless, exercise is". In the *Breviarium* it comes at the end of the Fulgentius extract. (These extracts are not continuous sections, but consist of several sentences strung together regardless of the connecting links between them.)

fuerit exercicium immoderate calefacit et desiccat, et ideo
eo vtantur moderate fleumatici. Quies vero humectat et
infrigidat, et hoc iuuat colericos. Reuera, vt naturales
dicunt, exercicium est vnum de alcioribus et nobilioribus
rebus que corpori humano possunt applicari in pro-
longacione vite et sue sanitatis regimine. Patet ergo ex
predictis quod exercicium est multum necessarium hominibus; supplebit enim fleobotomiam, farmaciam, atque
balneum, et cum hoc in exercicio non est timor nec
amaritudo neque expense, sed ibi est pura recreacio anime
et corporis dum tamen fiat per loca munda, quia tunc ex-
ponit se homo bono aeri, et gaudet in videndo longinqua
et propinqua et celum et maria atque viridia. Et in hiis
omnibus tenetur dominum deum suum commendare,
laudare, et magnificare. Bonum est igitur exercicium quia
hominem quodammodo vnit creatori suo.
   Species autem exerciciorum sunt multe secundum diuersitatem statuum et personarum. Aliqui enim sunt
fortes, aliqui debiles, aliqui diuites, aliqui pauperes, aliqui
prelati et honesti viri, aliqui religiosi et inclusi; et aliquando
est tempus pluuiale, et aliquando non. Et ideo oportet
multas habere species exerciciorum. Prima ergo et prin-
cipalis species exerciciorum est deambulare per loca alta
et munda, et est melior species inter omnes. Alius modus
exercicii est equitando, et iste modus est pro diuitibus.
Oportet autem quod prelati habeant alios exercitandi
modos. In camera igitur debet esse vna grossa corda in
fine nodata, et suspensa, et tunc accipiatur illa corda cum
duabus manibus, et homo debet stare erectus, ita quod non
tangat terram, et stet sic longo tempore: deinde saltabit
cum illa corda currendo quantum poterit, hinc inde se
voluendo et fortiter deambulando. Et si ludus iste non
placet ei, habeat lapidem de xxx librarum vbi sit anulus
infixus, et eum portet frequenter ab vna parte domus vsque

---

¹ MSS. note: "Galen, the Third Particula, Aphorisms: and ch. 1 of the
Regimen Sanitatis. Avicenna, *Canon*, Bk. 1" [Fen. 3].

moderate, it immoderately warms and dries the body, therefore let those who are phlegmatic of humour make a moderate use thereof. Repose, indeed, moistens and cools, and this is helpful to cholerics; but, nevertheless, exercise is, as the natural philosophers say, one of the highest and noblest things that can be applied to the human body for the prolongation of life, and the regulation of health.

It is evident, therefore, from what has been written, that exercise is very necessary to mankind, for it will serve as a complement to phlebotomy, pharmacy, and the bath; moreover, with exercise there is neither fear, nor distaste, nor expense; but pure recreation of soul and body when it is performed in the open; for then a man is exposed to wholesome air; and he rejoices in gazing far and near, and upon the sky, the sea and the green landscape; and he is therefore constrained to commend, to praise, and to magnify the Lord his God. Exercise therefore is good, since, in some measure, it unites a man to his Creator.[1]

There[2] are, however, many different kinds of exercise, according to the difference of rank and of persons. For some are strong, and some are weak; some are rich, and some are poor; some are prelates and men of rank, others are members of religious orders and are enclosed within their walls; moreover, the season is sometimes rainy, at other times it is fine. Therefore it is necessary to have several varieties of exercise. The first and most important of these is to walk abroad, choosing the uplands where the air is pure; this is the best of all. Riding is another form of exercise, but this is only for the wealthy. It behoves prelates,[3] however, to have some other method of taking exercise. Let such a man, therefore, have a stout rope, knotted at the end, hanging up in his chamber; and then, grasping the rope with both hands, let him raise himself up, and remain in that position for a long time without touching the ground; then, holding the rope and running with it as far as possible, let him jump into the air, turning himself round and round and strutting fiercely about. Or if this pastime does not please him, let him hold in his hands a stone, weighing thirty pounds, in which a ring has been fixed, and carry it about frequently from one part of his dwelling to another; or let him

[2] Here begins ch. VIII ("De Speciebus Exerciciorum") of B. de Gordonio, *Regimen Sanitatis*.
[3] In the *Florarium*, chapter "De Prelatis" (ch. 127), "prelates" are defined as including not only Bishops, etc. but all those comprised under the name of "Parsons". ("Episcopi Abbates et Priores et alii in sublimioribus ecclesie gradibus constituti et nonsolum isti dicuntur Prelati sed etiam illi qui secundum vulgare anglie appellantur *Parsone*").

ad aliam, vel teneat eundem lapidem superius in aere longo
tempore priusquam deponat, vel portet eum ad collum
suum vel inter manus. Et ita de aliis modis donec incipiat
fatigari; vel sic teneat baculum in manu sua, et alter
auferat sibi, si potest, recte trahendo, vel auferat denarium
a manu sua, et quod manus sit clausa. Alius autem modus
exercicii est quod retineat anelitum et quod impellat versus
capud vel versus ventrem; est multum vtile. Sunt etiam
alie species exercicii pro iuuenibus lasciuis, sicut currere,
luctari, et saltare, vel lapidem proicere, et ita de multis
aliis speciebus exerciciorum que iocando fiunt autem
iuuenibus. Et scire debes quod secundum omnes doctores
artis medicine exercicia corporalia[1] ante cibum voluntarie
et moderate facta custodiende sanitatis sunt perutilia.
Corporalia membra enim confortant, et superfluitates
humorum in eisdem existentium dissoluunt, calorem
naturalem confortant et ad digerendum adiuuant. Ideo
dicit Galienus, Cum exerciciis possumus humores super-
fluos dissoluere, et dissolutos purgare absque membrorum
nocumento. Quicumque, inquit, exercitantur, non necesse
est eis regulam diete obseruare, sed qui quieti sunt, die-
torum ordinem obseruare debent, cum corporis mundificacione, id est, fleobotomia, et farmacia, et huiusmodi.
Aque namque quando nimis quiescunt, putrescunt; similiter et ferrum et quodlibet metallum rubiginatur quando
minus debite vsitatur; sic et quies nimia in corporalibus
membris et sanguine humano malorum humorum est
generatiua nutritiua multiplicatiua et corrupcionis in-
ductiua. Sed dimittenda sunt exercicia fatigacione in-
chohante vel sudore apparente, Neque mox relicto exercicio manducent exercitati, nisi spacio quidem vnius hore
quiescant; deinde cibus sit paratus. Et statim cum incipiat
naturaliter esurire, cibum accipiat, et non ante; nec etiam
tunc tardet. Quoniam vt dicit Auicenna Stomachum
preter solitum pati famem putridis humoribus replet, nec
debet cibum sumere ad sacietatem, immo dimittere debet

[1] "temporalia" in MS. B.

hold this same stone up in the air for a long time before setting
it down, or lift it to his neck, or between his hands: the like
also with other methods of exercise, until he begins to tire: or
thus: let him hold a staff in his hand, and let another person,
pulling straight, try to drag it away from him, if he is able;
or let another strive to tear a penny from out of his closed hand.
Another method of taking exercise is to hold the breath and
impel it towards the head, or towards the belly, and this is
extremely useful. Other[1] forms of exercise are useful for playful
youths, such as running, wrestling, jumping, hurling stones, and
the many other sports in which young men should take delight.[2]

And it should be known that, according to all Doctors in the
Art of Medicine, moderate and voluntary exercise taken before
meals is most useful in preserving health, for it strengthens the
limbs and dissolves away the superfluity of humours existing in
them, increases the strength of the "natural heat", and aids
digestion. Therefore Galen says,

"By means of exercise we can dissolve the superfluous humours, and
then, having dissolved them, purge them away without harming the
limbs. Those", says he, "who take exercise, need not keep to a diet,
but those who are not thus occupied need both diet and such
bodily cleansing as phlebotomy, pharmacy and aids of a similar
nature."

For just as stagnant waters putrefy, and iron and every other
metal rusts from insufficient usage, so is excessive repose the
creator, nourisher, and multiplier of foul humours and the in-
ducer of corruption in the limbs of the body and in the human
blood. But exercise should be stopped with the onset of fatigue
or on the appearance of perspiration.

Nor should anybody commence to eat immediately after
exercise, but should rest for at least one hour, and then let their
food be prepared.[3] And let a man take food immediately he
begins to feel a natural hunger, and not before, nor let him then
delay, for, as Avicenna says,

The stomach, which is made to suffer hunger beyond its accustomed
length of time, becomes filled with putrefying humours, nor ought it
then to be glutted with food, but the meal should be finished whilst

[1] In the normal text of Bernardus de Gordonio (e.g. Sloane MS. 3097)
this sentence precedes the one describing the rope exercise. The extracts from
Bernardus temporarily cease at this point.
[2] Compare this with Fitz-Stephen's *Description of the young citizens sports in
Smithfield in the Twelfth Century*, ed. Lond. 1777, p. 47.
[3] The following extract is from B. de Gordonio: not, however, from
the *De Conservatione Vite Humane*, but from the *Lilium Medicine*, Particula v,
Chap. VIII.

cum appetitu. Quia satis cito postea cessabit appetitus.
Homines enim quibus donatur intellectus comedunt vt
viuant, sed quibus donatur sensualitas, viuere volunt vt
comedant. Nec accipiat in eadem mensa nihil nisi vnum
cibum; Et si amplius accipiat, minus malum est quando
subtile precedit grossum. Crudum non ponatur super semi-
coctum. Non accipiat lac et pisces in eadem mensa, neque
lac et vinum, quia disponunt ad lepram. Non accipiat
electuaria multum calida post cibum, nec etiam aliqua alia
multum calida, quoniam cibum corrumpunt in stomacho.
De quibusdam autem cibis versificator sic ait:

> Sunt nutritiue multum carnes vituline
> Est caro porcina sine vino peior ouina;
> Si tribuis vina tunc est cibus et medicina.
> Caseus et anguilla mortis cibus ille vel illa
> Ne bibas et rebibas et rebibendo bibas.
> Caseus et panis bonus est cibus et bene sanis.

Sed vt ait Isaac: Caseus est vniuersaliter pessimus
stomachi grauatiuus et difficilis digestionis, idcirco sepissime
illo vtentes colicam incidunt passionem, et in eorum reni-
bus lapides generantur. Similiter et capud debilitat et
subtilitatem ingenii perturbat. Sed magis vel minus nocet
propter diuersitatem sumendi. Quidam enim comedunt
illum ipso die quo fit, alii cum siccissimus fuerit et vetus.
Et nonnulli cum sit mediocris. Recens autem ceteris est
nutribilior et ventrem humefacit absque stomachi vllo
nocumento precipue si sale indigeat. Vetus vero est siccissimus, et cito in fumositatem et colericos conuertitur
humores. Talis enim caseus non est bonus ad nutriendum
corpus nec ad sanguinem bonum generandum nec ad ventrem humectandum. Caseus inter nouum et vetus mediocris satis est laudabilis vel illaudabilis secundum aliarum
predictarum extremitatum vicinitatem. Deuita, inquit,
omnem caseum, preter butirosum et pinguem de quo
parum commederi potest post commestionem. Sed loquens
quondam caseus seipsum veridica voce magnifice cepit

---

[1] This epigram is usually attributed to Socrates. (In the *Secret of Secrets*
it is ascribed to Hippocrates.)
[2] "Leprosy" at this period included almost all forms of skin disease.
[3] Here ends the extract from B. de Gordonio.
[4] *School of Salerno*, ll. 80, 73, 74, 90, 91, 103.

appetite remains, because the desire for food will cease quickly enough after that.

Men of intelligence eat in order that they may live, but sensualists wish to live in order that they may eat.[1] Let not more than one kind of food be taken at any one meal; but if more, however, is taken, it is less harmful when the light food precedes the heavy. Let not uncooked be taken on the top of half-cooked food. Do not take milk and fish at the same repast, nor milk and wine, for this disposes to leprosy.[2] Neither should very hot electuaries be taken after food, nor, for that matter, anything else which is very hot, for such corrupts the food which is in the stomach.[3]

The versifier thus speaks of various kinds of food:

[4]If thou on veal wilt dine, 'twill nourish well thy blood.
Pork without wine is worse than flesh of sheep as food;
Add wine to pork, 'tis then both food and physick good.
To eat an eel with cheese brings death within its train,
Unless thou drink, and drink, and drinking, drink again.
But cheese with bread is good, and will thy health maintain.

But, as Isaac[5] says,

"Cheese is universally the worst and most troublesome thing to the stomach, and most difficult to digest, and for that reason, those who take it frequently suffer from attacks of colic and develope stones in the kidneys. Similarly, it both confuses the head, and disturbs the clear working of the brain, but to a greater or less extent according to the manner in which it is taken; for some people eat it on the very day on which it is made, others when it is old and dry, and some when it is neither old nor new. Fresh cheese, is, however, more nourishing than other kinds, for it adds moisture to the belly without harming the stomach, especially if it contains no salt. Old cheese is extremely dry, and is quickly turned into vapour and colicky humours, and such cheese is neither good for nourishing the body, nor for forming good blood, nor for moistening the belly. Cheese, which is in a state somewhere between new and old, is to be commended or condemned according as it approximates to one or other of these two extremes." "Avoid", he says, "all cheese, except that containing a large proportion of butter and fat, of which kind a little may safely be taken after a good meal."

[6]Once upon a time, however, Cheese took upon himself to speak, and began to praise himself mightily with a truthful

---

[5] Isḥāḳ ibn Sulaimān or Isaac Judaeus (A.D. 830–940). The reference is to the chapter on cheese in his book on "Particular Diets". This extract on Cheese does not occur in Part xv of the *Breviarium*, but appears, together with the verses from the *School of Salerno*, as a separate Chapter "de Caseo" in Part xii.

[6] This is Mirfeld's method of introducing ll. 105 *et seq.* of the *School of Salerno*, where cheese is supposed to find its voice and speak for itself.

commendare, cuius dictis ego fiducialiter assensum prebeo
quia nunquam vt reor mentiebatur. Vnde et in diebus illis
aperiens os suum metrice sic loquens aiebat;

>Ignari medici me dicunt esse nociuum.
>Sed cum ignorent cur nocumenta feram.
>Expertis reor esse ratum, qua commoditate
>Languenti stomacho caseus addit opem.
>Caseus ante cibum confert, si defluat aluus.
>Si constipetur terminat ille dapes.
>Ad fundum stomachi dum sumpta cibaria crudant
>Vim Digestiuam non minus ille iuuat.
>Si¹ stomachus languet si quid minus appetit ille
>Fit gratis² stomacho consiliansque cibum.

Et ideo caseus insignis non est dandus nisi dignis.

>Caseus est carus sic dicit omnis auarus.
>Post pisces nuces, post carnes caseus aptus.

Preterea scire debes quod vinum bonum competit
temperate calidis quia coleram euacuat, et humidis quia
humiditatem temperat, et frigidis quia ad temperamentum
reducit, et siccis quia humectat et letificat. Et ita competit
omni complexioni, sed omni etati non competit; quoniam
dare vinum pueris est addere ignem igni secundum Auicennam. Et beatus Jeronimus, Vinum et adolescencia
duplex est incendium. Et quantum senes adiuuantur inde
tantum leduntur iuuenes secundum Galienum: sed vinum
temperate sumptum et secundum quod oportet, et quando
oportet, confortat multum scilicet virtutem vitalem naturalem et animalem et ideo summe letificat et audaciam inducit. Et quantum iuuat si temperate sumatur, tantum
et plus nocet si superflue bibatur, quoniam in stomacho
colerico conuertitur in coleram, in frigido in purum ace-
tum. Et ideo plerumque inducit in paralysim et spasmum.

---

¹ "si" in MSS. A and C and in *Brev*. Part XII. "sed" in B.
² "Gratus" in *Brev*. Part XII.

---

¹ *School of Salerno*, l. 114.
² The text now returns to excerpts from B. de Gordonio: *De Conservatione Vite Humane*, ch. XII, "De Potu Aque et Vini".
³ Not in the text of B. de Gordonio, which is resumed at "And Galen maintains".

voice (and I myself confidently agree with him, for I do not
think that he lied): wherefore, opening his mouth on that
occasion, he thus began to speak in rhyme:

Physicians who know naught ascribe great harm to me,
But yet they do not know why I can harmful be.
By those who wisest are I think 'tis understood
That cheese, if rightly used, to the weak stomach addeth good.
Cheese before food doth brace a relaxed stomach fast.
Let him that's constipated with cheese end his repast.
Cheese the digestion helps when food hath undigested lain
Within the stomach's depth; and when the stomach fain
Would flee from food, and languisheth, then cheese a boon is plain,
For by its aid the stomach doth digestive power regain.

Therefore cheese, good as it is, is not to be given but to those
with whom it agrees.

Thus saith the niggard; "Cheese is an expensive food".
"Nuts after fish; cheese after meat", such dieting is good.[1]

Moreover,[2] it should be known that wine of a good quality, if
moderately taken, agrees with those who are of a hot complexion, for it clears away their bile; likewise, it is helpful to
those who are moist of complexion, since it moderates their
humidity: similarly, it agrees with those who are cold since it
warms them back to a healthy mixture of the humours; and it
agrees also with those who are naturally dry, because it
moistens and gladdens. Thus it agrees with every complexion;
but it does not agree with all ages, for, according to Avicenna,
to give wine to children is to add flames to the fire. And the
Blessed St Jerome[3] says,

Wine and Youth make a twofold conflagration.

And Galen maintains that young men are injured by wine to
the same extent that the old are benefited by it. Wine, however,
if it is moderately and wisely taken at the right time, greatly
strengthens the vital, natural, and animal virtue,[4] and to a great
measure induces gladness and boldness. And by as much as it is
beneficial if moderately taken, to a greater extent it is harmful if
drunk to excess; for in a choleric stomach it is turned into bile, and
in a cold one into pure vinegar, and therefore it greatly tends
to paralysis and spasm.[5] Therefore, let him who is hot of com-

[4] The three fundamental faculties which, according to medieval ideas,
controlled the functioning of the digestive apparatus, brain, and heart.
[5] Here follows, in B. de Gordonio, a section on drunkenness, which the
priest John Mirfeld has curiously enough omitted. It includes the sentence
"Et ideo nullus catholicus scienter inebrietur". The quotation from the
chapter is resumed with the sentence commencing "Calidus ergo".

Calidus ergo de complexione sumat vinum album in colore
et subtile in substantia et cum temperata quantitate aque
quoniam iuuamenta vini non sunt nisi in corpore tem-
perato aut frigido. Non bibas vinum nouum quia multum
grauamen in corpore introducit; sed vinum si potes elige
citrinum in colore, mediocre in substantia, et odoriferum,
dictum in vulgari Prouincialium, Casteyn.[1] Hoc enim
vinum si temperate sumatur, tyriaca erit assumenti. Tante
siquidem nobilitatis est quod nichil malignum aggrauare
poterit corpus assumentis. Sicut enim vinum bonum est
altissima tyriaca cum sumitur sicut oportet, ita est letale
venenum cum sumitur sicut non oportet.

Potus ergo sit in mensa tua quanto minus erit possibile.
Hora autem comedendi, siue de die siue de nocte, est cum
aliquis incipit famescere, dum tum fames naturalis fuerit et
vera, et hoc intellige de illis qui habeant cibum paratum ad
libitum. Qui autem non habeant, comedant quando habere
potuerint, quia tales non subiacent legibus artis huiusmodi.

Preterea sciendum est iuxta doctrinam, scilicet, Galieni
in Regimine Sanitatis quod in eadem mensa nunquam
competunt cibaria plura, et ideo ipse Galienus erat con-
tentus in mane solo pane et in sero solis carnibus; quando
autem duo cibaria sumuntur in eadem mensa, tunc malum
est in se, et malum est in relacione vnius ad alterum.
In se, quoniam aliter laborat natura in digerendo grossa,
aliter in digerendo subtilia, et ita de aliis qualitatibus[2] ci-
borum. Similiter malum est in relacione, quoniam si cibus
subtilis precedat, cito digeritur, et trahit secum grossum in-
digestum. Quod si grossus precedat, tunc subtilis, cum erit

---

[1] *Sic* in MSS. A, C and D. "Castym" in B. Omitted in E and F.
[2] "quantitatibus" in C.

---

[1] "Called 'Chestnut' by the Provençals." This is an addition by Mirfeld.
"Province" wine was regularly imported into England at this period.
Concerning this wine (which he does not name) B. de Gordonio adds: "And
understand that when we speak of wine we mean the best; namely, not white
wine nor thin or weak or light green wine such as is cultivated in France

plexion, drink a wine which is white in colour and light in body, and let it be taken with a moderate amount of water, for wine is beneficial in effect only upon a temperate or cold body. Do not drink new wine, for it is most detrimental to the body; but, if possible, choose a wine which is light yellow in colour, medium in body, and fragrant in bouquet, and which is colloquially termed "Chestnut" by the inhabitants of Provence;[1] for such wine, if moderately taken, will be as beneficial to the drinker as the finest tyriac.[2] Indeed, so excellent in quality is this wine that it can do no harm to whoever takes it in moderation. Just as good wine, however, can be the finest antidote[3] when taken as it should be, so too can it be a most deadly poison when taken in the opposite manner. Let thy drink at meals be as little as possible.

[4]The time, however, to take food, whether by day or by night, is when anyone begins to feel hungry, and when the hunger is natural and genuine; and this applies only to those who can have their food prepared to their desire, but let those who cannot do so, dine whenever they are able, for such are not subject to these laws.

[5]Moreover, it should be known that, according to the doctrine of Galen, in the *Regimen of Health*, several kinds of food should not be taken at the same meal; and therefore Galen himself was content to eat only bread in the morning and meat at the setting of the sun. When, however, two kinds of food are taken at one meal, then it is both bad in itself, and bad in the relation of the one food to the other. It is bad in itself, since Nature works one way in digesting heavy foods, and along different lines in digesting light foods, and so on concerning other kinds of food. Similarly, it is bad with regard to the relationship; for if the light food is taken first, it will be speedily digested and carry along with it the heavy food before the digestion of the

[i.e. Old France] and in the mountains; nor Greek [? Chian] wine, nor wine from La Marche [i.e. modern La Creuse, in France], or Cyprus, and neither old wine nor new, but light yellow...such as commonly comes from the districts around Montpellier [where Bernard was medical professor] and in fact from all over the province of Narbonne [which, at the date of the composition of these remarks (i.e. 1307) formed part o Provence]."

[2] The universal panacea, theriaca. The word also means "antidote".
[3] Presumably used here in its sense of "antidote" as opposed to the "deadly poison". Our author is fond of puns. This sentence is apparently his own.
[4] The following paragraph is from the *Regimen Sanitatis* of Particula v of B. de Gordonio's *Lilium Medicine*.
[5] Here begins an extract from the chapter "De Ordine Cibi" of B. de Gordonio, *De Conservatione Vite Humane*, Chap. XI.

digestus, corrumpetur, quia non habebit exitum. Et ideo quocumque istorum modorum fiet, semper erit malum, sed magis malum est quando subtilis sequatur. Quoniam corrupcio nunquam rectificatur per subsequencia, Quoniam mutacio est facta ad aliam[1] speciem, sed cruditas est citra speciem. Et ideo quodammodo rectificabile est, minus ergo malum est quando subtilis precedit, et in hoc conueniunt Auicenna et Galienus. Sane autem intelligendum est quod stomachus duas habet partes, superiorem videlicet, et inferiorem. Superior[2] enim pars carnosa est et calida, inferior autem panniculosa per quam fit appetitus. Nunc autem si cibus grossus esset in profundo cum haberet obiectum proporcionale digeretur grossum per fortem calorem. Et quia subtilis cibus non indiget forti calore, ideo conuenienter vt apparet esset subtilis cibus in parte superiori stomachi et ita bona esset proporcio.

Quare grossum vt videtur deberet precedere, sed quia exquisite Natura stomachi cognosci non potest nec quantitatem offerendorum certis litteris denotare possumus, ideo in statera cibum stomacho proporcionabilem secundum superius et inferius ponere nequiuimus, nec certitudinem de hoc habere possumus, neque ex parte stomachi neque ex

[1] "Illam" in B.
[2] *Sic* in all MSS. for "Inferior", etc. (see note to translation).

---

[1] Not in the *Breviarium*. The MSS. of the *Florarium* all say exactly the opposite to the standard B. de Gordonio text (of which Sloane MS. 3097 in the British Museum, which was written in France in A.D. 1311 i.e. only four years after the completion of the *Regimen* of Bernardus, has been taken as the example). Bernardus says that the lower part is fleshy and the upper is stringy and cold. It is, however, unlikely that Mirfeld would diametrically oppose such an authority whom he quotes so fully, and that too, without assigning a reason, and especially as the Bernard version is indicated as being the correct one by what follows. Unfortunately this passage occurs only in A, B, C and D, but as all the MSS. are corrupt, the presumption is that Mirfeld actually followed Bernardus, but that an early transcriber fell into the error of leaving out part of the sentence, and that subsequent copyists followed the incorrect version. It is difficult to state precisely how much Bernardus knew about the stomach. He evidently means the oesophagus when he speaks of the "upper", and the stomach proper, when he speaks of the "lower" part; but he has perhaps misread Constantinus Africanus, and has confused the upper and lower *orifice* of the stomach with the inner and outer coat as explained by that

latter has been completed. If, however, the heavy food is eaten first, then the light food, when digested, will become corrupted, because it will have no way of escape. Therefore whichever of these methods is followed, the result will always be evil, but more so when the light food follows the heavy, for the corruption is never subsequently set right; for in the case of the light food, the change into putrefaction has already taken place, whereas, in the case of the heavy undigested food, the process stops short of this point. Therefore, to whatever extent this evil is remediable, it is less evil when the light food precedes the heavy food, and in this opinion both Avicenna and Galen agree.

It can be reasonably understood that the stomach has two parts, the upper, namely, and the lower. The upper part is fleshy and hot, whilst the lower is composed of membranes, and is where the appetite is generated.[1] Now if the heavy food were to be sent to the lowest part of the stomach, it would find itself in the neighbourhood of the greater proportion of the natural heat of the stomach, and it would thus be digested by this powerful heat.[2] And because the light food does not require very much heat in order to digest it, therefore it would appear to be the best plan that the lighter food should be in the upper part of the stomach, and thus everything would be in the correct proportion. Wherefore it would seem that the heavy food ought to be eaten before the light: but since the nature of the stomach cannot be accurately known, nor can we state in fixed terms the amount of different kinds of food to be given; nor can we strike a balance as to the proportion of food that is to be sent to the upper or lower part of the stomach; since neither can we attain to any certainty as to this, either with regard to the stomach or to the food; it behoves us therefore to

writer. Galen dissected animals, and so did the medievals; it is, however, difficult to ascertain how far the knowledge of Bernardus extended. He seems to have suspected, although not to have been fully conversant with, the peristaltic action of the oesophagus; for he says—in the *Lilium Medicine* (Particula v, c. 2, "De Debilitate Appetitus")—that in the case of certain Jews, hung up by the heels, the food given ascended to the stomach, showing that this organ possessed the power of attracting food to itself! Constantinus held that the food fell straight down the oesophagus into the stomach, presumably in the way that water falls when poured into a well.

[2] According to medieval theory (see p. 31), digestion of the food in the stomach was produced by the innate heat from the liver cooking it, as it were, in a cauldron. Since flesh was regarded as "hot" in this sense, it follows that food at the bottom (*not* the modern "fundus") of the stomach, being in the fleshy part and nearer to the liver, would be in the region of the greatest heat. "Heavy" food is meat, etc.; "light" food, poultry, milk, etc.

parte cibi. Quare oportet sequi minus periculosam viam, videlicet, quod subtile precedat vt predictum est. Et in hoc conueniunt omnes doctores huius facultatis: Sed nos Anglici ex longissima consuetudine oppositum tenemus. Et ideo forte nobis via illa vtilissima reputatur. Quia consuetudo vt dicitur est altera natura, id est, alterat naturam.

Sed caue ne comedas donec certissime noueris stomachum esse vacuum a priori cibo, quod cognosces per desiderium comedendi et per superfluitatem saliue decurrentis ad os; quia si quis cibum sumpserit absque corporis necessitate, id est, sine comedendi desiderio, cibus tunc inueniet calorem naturalem stomachi gelidum. Si vero cum desiderio sumpserit cibum inueniet calorem naturalem sicut incensum. Et ideo cum incipis comedendi habere desiderium debes statim comedere, quia nisi tunc cito comederis statim implebitur stomachus pessimis humoribus et turbabitur cerebrum vapore pessimo, Et cum postea apponitur cibus fit stomachi virtus tepidus et illis humoribus corruptus et non proficit corpori quod sumitur; ideo versificator sic ait:

> Tu nunquam comedas stomachum nisi noueris ante
> Purgatum vacuumque cibo quem sumpseris ante.

Post cibum autem quiescas stando vel paulatim deambulando. Quia omnis fortis motus post prandium corrumpit cibum et virtus digestiua viget per quietam.

Sompnus tamen meredianus sit aliquando nullus semper exiguus autem iuxta illud.

> Sit breuis aut nullus sompnus tibi meredianus.

Et secundum quod vult Auicenna, Sani debent melius comedere circa noctem quam in mane. Quia circa noctem calor naturalis clauditur interius et circa viscera congregatur. Fleumatici tamen non multum frigidi quia pauco indigent exercicio ad paucum calorem excitandum de die

---

[1] End of this extract from B. de Gordonio.
[2] It is hardly possible to reproduce the pun on "alter" in the translation.

follow the less dangerous path, namely, to take the lighter food first, as has already been said.[1] And in this all the doctors of the faculty agree; but we English, from long custom, hold the opposite opinion; and therefore, perchance by us that way is considered the best, because, as it is said, "Habit is second nature", that is, it provides us with another nature.[2]

[3] But beware that thou dine not until thou knowest within thyself that the stomach is free of the food which has been previously taken: and this will be known by the desire to eat, and by the superfluity of saliva running down into the mouth. For, if anybody partakes of food when there is no real necessity for so doing, that is, when there is no desire to eat, then the food will find the natural heat of the stomach cooled: but when a person eats with a true desire to do so, then the food will find the natural heat to be, as it were, kindled. Therefore, when thou shalt begin to desire food, thou shouldest immediately eat, for if thou dost not do so, then the stomach will be immediately filled with foul humours, and the brain troubled with impure vapours: and although food should be afterwards placed before thee, yet the virtue of the stomach has been made lukewarm, and is corrupted by those humours, and therefore the food will not bring any benefit to the body of him who takes it. Therefore the versifier thus says:

[4] Thou shouldst not dine until within thou feel
The stomach to be freed from all its former meal.

After food, however, rest awhile, either standing up or walking about a little, for all violent movement after meals corrupts the food; moreover the digestive virtue flourishes on repose. Let thy midday sleep, however, according to that same poem, be always little and sometimes none at all.

[5] Quite short, else none, for thee, thy midday sleep should be.

And, as Avicenna maintains,[6]

Healthy men ought to dine rather towards night time than in the morning,

for then the natural heat is shut up within the body, and gathered about the viscera. Phlegmatics, however, ought not to eat much that is cold during the course of a day, since they

---

[3] A return is made to the extracts from the *Secret of Secrets*.
[4] *School of Salerno*, ll. 22–24.
[5] *Ibid.* l. 15.
[6] The treatise on food is in Part II of Avicenna's *Cantica*.

debent comedere, et post suaue exercicium quiescere. Et addit versificator sic dicens

Lote cale sta pasce vel hii, frigesce minute.

Et intellige quod nullus debet sumere cibum post exercicium vel balneum nisi prius fuerit quietatus, et tunc cum prandere volueris, si diues sis ponantur ante te cibi multi et quos desiderat anima tua comede. Si enim sunt duo cibaria quorum vnum est optimum et aliud est minus bonum, Si tunc minus bonum desideratur et appetitur, talis cibus debet cicius sumi quam alter melior in natura sua. Quoniam quod melius sapit melius nutrit secundum Auicennam, et ratio dictorum est, quoniam cibus qui accipitur cum delectacione auide amplectitur a stomacho et comprehenditur et diu retinetur, et ideo melius digeritur. Et ille qui melius digeritur, melius est corpori iuuatiuus. Alter autem qui non appetitur sumitur cum quodam fastidio et ideo non ita bene digeritur. Si ergo plus appeteret carnes mutouinas quam gallinas, mutouine tunc essent concedende, et sic autem de aliis. Sed vbi est multa distancia in qualitate cibariorum, non est ita procedendum. Et nota quod humana complexio si sit temperata cum consimilibus debet conseruari. Si vero distemperata fuerit per contrarium reducatur paulatim ad temperamentum.

Scias preterea quod omnia accidencia anime desiccant excepto gaudio quod humectat. Quedam etiam calefaciunt velud ira vnde et confert melancolicis nocet vero colericis.

Item

Cena breuis vel cena leuis fit raro molesta,
Magna nocet, medicina docet, res est manifesta.

Et hoc manifeste verum est nisi in quibusdam qui longa consuetudine excusantur qui magnam vim habent, et hoc quidem experimento cognoscimus. Quoniam aliqui con-

---

[1] *School of Salerno*, l. 14.
[2] Bernardus de Gordonio again. Section "De Tempore sumendi cibum" and "De Cibo Desiderato" (*De Conservatione Vite Humane*).

require a little exercise to induce a little heat, and they ought to rest after a light exercise. And the versifier thus adds:

Fresh from the bath get warm; having dined, stand or walk; get cool by degrees.[1]

And[2] understand that nobody ought to take food after exercise or the bath, unless he shall have first rested, and then, when thou wilt, dine. And if thou art rich, and many kinds of food are placed before thee, then take that which thy soul desireth. If, however, there are but two foods, both of which are good, but one of which is excellent from the dietetic point of view, the other not quite so good, and if the latter is desired and longed for, then it should be taken in preference to the former; for that which tastes better nourisheth better, according to Avicenna, and the reason of this remark is that the food which is taken with delight is eagerly embraced by the stomach, and is gripped and retained by it for a long time, and therefore it is better digested, and that which is better digested is more helpful to the body. The other food, for which there is no desire, is taken with a certain amount of aversion, and is therefore not so well digested. If, then, mutton should be desired in preference to poultry, a concession should be made, and the former should be eaten, and thus of other kinds of food. Where, however, there is a considerable difference in the quality of the foods, this method is not to be followed. And mark thou that the human "complexion", if it is "temperate", should be preserved by taking foods of a similar complexion; and if it is not temperate,[3] it should be gradually brought back to the healthy state by means of foods which are opposite in nature to that of its prevailing humour.

[4]It should be known, moreover, that all mental disturbances dry up the body, except Joy, which moistens it. Some even raise its heat, as for example, Rage, which therefore works a welcome change in melancholics, but is harmful to cholerics. Thus:

[5]Supper light or brief doth rarely health molest,
Heavy bringeth grief; 'tis Medicine's law, and manifest.

[6]And this is manifestly true, except in the case of those who have obtained a dispensation by reason of long habit, or those who possess great strength. And this we know, indeed, by ex-

---

[3] That is, healthy: the maintenance of the healthy, or temperate, complexion by procuring the correct proportion of the humours. This was effected by "treating with opposites", that is, in giving to those who were too "cold" such food as was considered to be "hot", e.g. wine.

[4] Perhaps based upon B. de Gordonio, *Ibid.* chap. "De Accidentibus Animae".

[5] *School of Salerno.* De Renzi, ll. 184, 185.

[6] B. de Gordonio, *Ibid.* chap. "De Consuetudine".

sueuerunt comedere quater in die et non leduntur et
aliqui consueuerunt vigilare de nocte et dormire de die, et
aliqui consueuerunt comedere fabas et carnes bouinas
antiquas, et aliqui vulpes et alia huiusmodi innumerabilia,
et tamen dicunt se esse sanissimos et bene se habentes. Et
propter hoc dicebat Galienus, Consuetudo etas et complexio indigent similibus, magnam ergo vim habet consuetudo et non solum hoc est manifestum per viam experi-
menti et per auctoritates immo etiam per rationes.
Quoniam vt predictum est natura gaudet in consueto et in
eo delectatur. Et ideo dixit Auicenna quod experimentum
in hoc vincit rationem. Quoniam, inquit, malus cibus
vsitatus melior est bono non vsitato. Oppositum tamen
omnium istorum videtur dicere Constantinus cum ait, Non
gaudeant malo cibo vtentes quoniam si non in presenti
leduntur in posterum percussionem non euadunt. Et ideo
tucius est talem consuetudinem remouere sed tamen non
subito sed paulatim vt dando a principio illa cibaria mala
et parum de bonis et sic paulatim augere bona et mala
diminuere. Quoniam licet videatur eis quod bene se
habere racione etatis vel temporis aut fortitudinis virtutis
vel etiam ratione consuetudinis, nichilominus paulatim
cadunt virtutes in mineris et quotidie parant se ad lepram
aut ad paralysim et ydropisym siue ad mortem subitaneam,
Sicut et illi qui parum dormiunt aut qui nimis excitant se
post cibum, aut qui summa mensura sustinent calorem vel
frigus, et ita de multis aliis consimilibus. Vere de talibus
dicit Constantinus quod percussionem non euadent; licet
enim quantum est de presenti omnibus talibus videatur
quod conferant et bene ferant, nichilominus tamen in
interioribus sunt corrupti, et ideo paulatim sunt reducendi
vt predictum est, quia licet consuetudo sit tenenda, si
conueniat cum naturalibus, omnis tamen consuetudo in-
naturalis reducenda est ad naturalem. Vt ergo omnia predicta euadas incommoda viue in abstinencia. Omnium
enim medicinarum secundum Galienum sublimior est Abs-

perience. For some people are accustomed to dine four times a
day, and yet are not harmed by it; others stay up at night and
sleep during the day; others eat beans and tough and ancient
beef; and some eat foxes and innumerable things of that
nature; and yet they say that they are most healthy and keep
well, and for this reason Galen[1] used to say,

Custom, age, and complexion, need foods which are in agreement
with them; Therefore custom is very strong; and this is manifest not
only by proof, but also by authority, and even by reason; for, as has
been said before, Nature takes pleasure in that to which she is accustomed, and delights in it.

And as Avicenna says,

"In this case experience conquers reason. For", says he, "bad food
to which you are used is better than good food to which you are not
accustomed."

Constantinus [Africanus], however, would seem to be in
opposition to all of these writers, when he says,

Let not those who take bad food rejoice, for although they are not
harmed at the time, they cannot ultimately escape the blow of fate.

And therefore it is safer to change such a habit; but not, however, suddenly, but little by little, at first taking the bad foods
with a little of the good, and gradually increasing the good, and
diminishing the bad. And although they seem to be healthy by
reason of their age, the season, or the strength of their constitution, and even by reason of their habits, yet nevertheless their
reserves of strength fall away from them little by little, and
they daily qualify themselves for leprosy, paralysis, dropsy, or
even sudden death. In such a case, too, are those who do not
sleep much, or who take immoderate exercise after meals, or
suffer heat or cold in great degree, and thus of many others who
act similarly. Truly Constantinus says of these that they cannot
escape. For although apparently they are permitted to thrive
and to keep well for the present, nevertheless, of a truth, they
are corrupted away in their inward parts, and therefore must
be brought back to a sane method of living by the gradual
means described above. For although a habit is permissible if
it is in accordance with nature, every unnatural habit must be
changed into a natural one. Therefore, live in abstinence, in
order to avoid all the aforesaid harm. For according to
Galen,

Of all medicines the most sublime is abstinence, and gluttony kills
more men than the sword.

[1] MSS. note, *De Ingeniis*, cap. vIII (more commonly known as the *Methodus
Medendi*, or *Therapeutika*).

tinencia,[1] Et plures interficit gula quam gladius.[1] Et Beda
in quadam opera sic ait, Qui precepta contempnit medici
de vita periclitatur vt predictum est. Sed forte loquitur ibi
de medico spirituali, loquens enim de medicis corporalibus[2]
ait beatus Ambrosius, Contraria condicioni diuine precepta sunt medicine, A ieiunio enim reuocant, lugubrare
non sinunt, et ab omni intencione meditationis abducunt.
Vnde qui se medicis dederit seipsum sibi abnegat; expro-
bando enim dicitur de Asa rege Iuda qui egrotauit dolore
pedum vehementissime, Nec etiam in infirmitate sua que-
siuit dominum, sed magis in medicorum arte confisus est,
vnde et mortuus est. Ideo Salomon ait, Etenim neque
herba neque malagma sanauit infirmos, sed tuus domine
sermo, qui omnia sanat. Tu es domine qui vite et mortis
habes potestatem, et deducis ad portas mortis et reducis.
Sana me ergo domine et sanabor; saluum me fac et saluus
ero, quoniam laus mea tu es domine deus meus. Amen.

---

[1] The two sentences run in this order in MSS. A, C and D, but reversed
in B.

[2] *Sic* in MSS. A and C. "spiritualibus" in B.

And Bede thus speaks in a certain work,

He who despises the injunctions of the physician, goes in peril of his life,

as has already been said. But perhaps he is speaking there of the spiritual physician, for speaking of physicians of the body, the blessed St Ambrose[1] says,

The precepts of Medicine are opposed to the Divine Command, for they recall men from fasting, they do not allow them to indulge in grief, and they divert them from all thought of meditation. Therefore he who gives himself over to the physicians, abnegates his personality.

In proof of which it is said of Asa King of Judah, that when he was most gravely stricken with disease[2] in his feet, he did not even so seek out the Lord in his infirmity; but trusted more in the skill of the physicians; wherefore he died. Therefore Solomon says,[3]

For it was neither herb nor mollifying plaster that restored the sick to health; but thy word, O Lord, which healeth all things. Thou art the Lord who hast power of life and death; and thou leadest to the gates of death, and bringest back again.[4] Heal me therefore, O Lord, and I shall be healed; save me, and I shall be saved: for thou art my praise, O Lord my God. Amen.

[1] Archbishop of Milan. The reference is to his Exposition of Psalm 118.
[2] Vulgate. II Chronicles, ch. 16, v. 12.
[3] Vulgate. Wisdom of Solomon, ch. 16, vv. 12 and 13.
[4] Vulgate. Jeremiah, ch. 17, v. 14.

IV. EPILOGUE

FLORARIUM BARTHOLOMEI

Terminando iam opusculum quod incepi quodque deo adiuuante peregi vt potui immensas deo omnipotenti gratiarum refero acciones. Vereor iam prorsus ne aut grandia minus digne tractasse inueniar aut pertractata amplioribus superflue pertractasse. Sicubi igitur in hac compilacione deuiaui parcatur michi quia ignorans feci. Vbi vero recte processi laudetur gratia Christi Qui asino quondam inueniri prestitit humano vti eloquio. Lege ergo illam primo Karissime frater si placet solus et corrige. Ne si proferatur in medium non emendata magis forte compilatoris publicetur temeritas quam caritas lectoris edificetur. Quod si palam fieri vtile probaueris tunc si quid in ea quod ad me pertinuit minus competenter prolatum vel ordinatum reperieris non sit tibi pigrum aut per temetipsum emendare aut michi resignare emendandum. Si fraudari non vis illa promissione sapientie increate qua ait Qui elucidant me vitam eternam habebunt.

Scio vtique quod hec mea impolita operacio a multis litterarum scientia tumidis despicietur atque subsauciabitur. Indignabuntur enim contra me cur ego Ydiota et pene nichil sciens presumpserim tale aliquid aggredi. Sed quid queso in hoc deliqui aut quid mali feci doctrinam scribens sanctorum et verba recitans virorum iustorum?

Sed ex hoc forte scandalizabuntur multi quod huic compilacioni certum nomen imposui: sed si cacco meo et cani meo nomen absque calumpnia possum imponere quare non etiam et quaterno meo? Obtenebratum est vtique insipiens cor eorum, excecauit enim eos malicia eorum. Sed ablatrent licet et a tergo mordeant inuidi et dolosi ego prorsus non curo. Testis enim meus in hac parte de in-

EPILOGUE

FLORARIUM BARTHOLOMEI

In terminating this little work which I took in hand, and which, with God's help, I have carried through to the best of my ability, immense is the gratitude which I offer to Almighty God. I fear, indeed truly, lest I may be found to have dealt with sublime things in too unworthy a manner, or that those matters which have been given fuller treatment will be found to have received undue attention. So wherever in this compilation I shall be found to have gone astray, let it be forgiven me since I have erred in ignorance; and for whatever I have done aright let praise be given to the grace of Christ, who once preferred to be found riding upon an ass rather than avail Himself of human speech. Therefore, Dearest Brother, be so good as to read this book through first by yourself, and correct it; lest by publication in an uncorrected state, it may perchance serve to demonstrate the temerity of the compiler rather than to develope the charity of the reader. But if you should decide that it should be made publicly useful, then should you find therein anything which, so far as my own work is concerned, is not well enough set forth or arranged, do not be averse either to correcting it yourself or to returning it to me for correction, if you do not wish to lose that promise of Increate Wisdom which says, "Those who make me understood shall have everlasting life".[1]

I know, assuredly, that this inelegant work of mine will be despised and torn in pieces by many of those who are puffed up with their literary skill; and they will wax indignant against me, because I, uninstructed in Theology and almost ignorant of it, have dared to embark upon such a task: but what, I ask, have I done amiss, or what evil have I committed, in writing down the doctrine held by the saints and in reciting the words of righteous men?

Many perchance will be scandalised because I have called this compilation by such a title as *Florarium Bartholomei*; but if I am permitted to give a name to my cat or my dog without receiving abuse, why not also to my book?

For their foolish heart is darkened; their malice hath blinded them.[2]

Let the envious and deceitful men bark, however, and although they bite at me from behind, I truly do not care, for

---

[1] Vulgate, Ecclesiasticus, ch. 24, v. 31.
[2] Vulgate, Romans, ch. 1, v. 21; Wisdom, ch. 2, v. 21.

tentione mea in celis est. Et ideo non timebo quid faciat
mihi homo. Sed humiliter te deposco karissime frater et
omnes alios in quorumcumque manus catholicorum compilacio ista ex multis et diuersis doctorum ortodoxorum
sentenciis contexta deuenerit quatinus pro me peccatore
ad deum omnipotentem preces porrigere velitis vt inter-
cessione eius gloriosissimi apostoli sancti Bartholomei et
vestrarum precum interuentu antiquitus ego peccator
priscis depositis delictorum inuolucris in nouum reuiuiscam
hominem et modicum illud quod iam restat de vite mee
termino ad gloriosissimi eius nominis honorem et anime
mee vtilitatem in caritate eius perfecta et sacratissimorum
mandatorum eius vera et humili obediencia valeam con-
summare et vt omni meorum a deo percepta Venia peccatorum et emendacione a sorde facinorum ad celi gaudia
omnibus veris Christicolis repromissa Vna vobiscum valeam
peruenire vbi cum patre et spiritu sancto regnat dominus
deus noster Ihesus Christus dei filius benedictus. In cuius
nomine flectitur omne genu celestium terrestrium et in-
fernorum Cui est honor et gloria virtus et magnificencia
potestas regnum et imperium per infinita seculorum secula.
Amen.

Explicit liber qui intitulatur Florarium Bartholomei Deo
gracias Opere completo sit laus et gloria Christo.

concerning my intention in this matter, my witness is in Heaven; "therefore I shall not fear what man may do unto me":[1] but I humbly beseech you, Dearest Brother, and all those other true Catholics, into whose hands shall come this compilation (consisting as it does of many and various words of orthodox Doctors) that, as much as you are willing to grant me, you will pray for me (a sinner) to Almighty God; so that, through the intercession of His most glorious Apostle St Bartholomew, and the intervention of your own prayers, I, steeped in sin from of old as I am, may cast aside the former fetters of my misdeeds, and may be made into a new man: and that the little of life that is left me I may be enabled to complete to the honour of His most glorious Name and to the advantage of my own soul, in His perfect love, and by true and humble obedience to His most Holy commands; and that I, fully and previously pardoned by God of all my sins, and purified from the filthiness of my misdeeds, may attain with you to those joys promised in Heaven to all true followers of Christ; where with God the Father and the Holy Spirit reigneth the Blessed Son of God, our Lord God Jesus Christ, at whose Name every knee doth bow in Heaven, Earth, and Hell; to whom be Honour and Glory, Might, Majesty and Power, Dominion, and Empire, for ever and ever. Amen.

Here endeth the book called *Florarium Bartholomei*. Thanks be to God, and praise and glory be to Christ, for the completion of the work.

[1] Vulgate, Psalm 55, v. 11.

164

To indicate the nature of the contents of the *Florarium,*
the titles of the 175 chapters of which it is composed are
printed below.

Proemium
De Abstinencia
 Begins: Abstinencia est statu-
  tum prandendi tempus non
  preuenire
De Accidia
De Adulacione
De Adulterio
De Amatoribus Mundi
De Ambicione
De Amore Dei
De Angelis
De Antichristo
De Auaricia
De Baptismo
De Blasphemia
De Bonitate Dei
De Breuitate humane vite
De Caritate
De Castitate
De Celebracione Missarum
De Cogitacionibus Prauis
De Confessione Peccatorum
De Compunccione
De Consciencia
De Consilio Bono
De Consuetudine
De Conuiuiis
De Corpore Christi
De Correccione Fraterna
De Crapula
De Cruce Christi
De Curiositate
De Dampnatis
De Decimis
De Deliciis
De Desperacione
De Detraccione
De Deuocione
De Die Iudicii
De Dileccione Inimici
De Dileccione Parentum
De Dileccione Proximi
De Discrecione
De Diuiciis
De Diuiniis Officiis
De Duricia Cordis
De Ebrietate
De Elemosina
De Excommunicacione
De Extrema Vnccione
De Festiuitatibus
De Fide
De Filio Dei
De Fletu
De Fortitudine
De Gaudiis Celi
De Gaudio Spirituali
De Gracia
De Graciarum Accione
De Gula

De Humana Laude
De Humilitate
De Iactancia
De Ieiunio
De HOC NOMINE IHESUS
De Ignorancia
De Inani Gloria
De Incarnacione Christi
De Indigne siue Quotidie cele-
  brantibus
De Indulgencia Delinquencium
De Indulgenciis
De Indumentis
De Ingratitudine
De Inuidia
De Ipocrisi
De Ira
De Iudicio
De Iuramentis
De Iusticia
De Labore Manuum
De Laude Dei
De Leccione
De Loquacitate
De Luxuria
De Malediccione
De Mandatis Dei
De Mansuetudine
De Maria Virgine Gloriosa
De Martirio
De Matrimonio
De Medicis et eorum Medicinis
De Meditacione Sancta
De Mendacio
De Mendicitate
De Miseria Condicionis Humane
De Misericordia
De Monachis et Regularibus
De Morte Temporali
De Mortificacione Carnis
De Mulieribus
De Mundanis Honoribus
De Muneribus
De Natiuitate Christi
De Necligencia
De Negociis Secularibus
De Nobilitate Generis
De Obediencia
De Occulto Dei Iudicio
De Ociositate
De Occupacione Bona
De Odio Proximorum
De Operibus Misericordie
De Oracione
De Pace
De Paciencia
De Paradyso
De Passione Christi
De Paupertate
De Peccatis Mortalibus
De Peccatis Venialibus

De Peccato In Spiritum Sanc-
  tum
De Penis Inferni
De Penitencia
De Perseuerancia
De Pollucione Nocturna
De Praua Societate
De Preciositate Temporis
De Predicacione
De Predicatoribus
De Prelatis
De Presumpcione
De Primis Motibus
De Prosperitate
De Psalmis
De Prudencia
De Purgatorio
De Residiuacione
De Redempcione generis Hu-
  mani
De Religione Christiana
An Relinquenda sunt Omnia
De Resurreccione Mortuorum
De Sacerdotibus
De Sacramentis in generali
De Sanctis
De Sapiencia
De Scandale
De Securitate
De Sera Conuersione ad Deum
De Silencio
De Symonia
De Sobrietate
De Societate Bona
De Solitudine
De Solicitudine
De Sompnis
De Sompno
De Sortilegio
De Spe
De Spiritu Sancto
De Superbia
De Suspicione Mala
De Temerario Iudicio
De Temptacione
De Temptantibus Deum
De Timore Domini
De Tribulacione
De Trinitate Sancta
De Tristicia
De Vana Leticia
De Verbis Ociosis
De Veritate
De Vigilia
De Vita Actiua
De Vita Contemplatiua
De Vita Perfecta
De Voluntate Bona
De Voto
De Vsura
Terminacio operis (Epilogue)

Appendices

APPENDICES A AND B

GENERAL NOTES ON THE PREPARATION OF THE TEXTS USED IN THIS EDITION

The Latin text of the MSS. is written in the abbreviated form usual in the Middle Ages. This has been transcribed in full, transcription being as literal as possible, and the usual medieval spelling retained (for instance in the use of *u* and *v* and of certain of the capitals). The modern system of capital lettering has been adopted as far as possible; and punctuation and paragraphing have been supplied to render the work more intelligible. Marginal notes in the Latin MSS., where they occur, are incorporated in the Notes to the Translation.

It should be noted that the quotations from the *School of Salerno* are not written out as verse in any of the MSS. The words of each line follow each other as prose, without any other indication as to their nature except for the marginal note "verses". It has, however, been thought advisable, for the sake of clarity and facility of reference, to disinter them, and to establish them apart in the enjoyment of the full dignity attendant upon poetical quotation.

APPENDIX A

NOTES ON THE MSS. USED FOR THE TEXT OF THE *BREVIARIUM BARTHOLOMEI*

(1) *Pembroke College, Oxford, MS. No. 2.*

A late fourteenth-century MS. containing 359 folios, and in its ancient binding. The only copy containing the *Sinonoma Bartholomei* (edited by Mowat). In addition to this and to the text of the work itself, it has the astronomical Calendar of John Somer, composed in 1380, the "Quid pro Quo", and the section on "Weights and Measures" printed in this work. The MS. formerly belonged to the Hospital of St John the Baptist attached to Abingdon Abbey, and is illuminated with a miniature of the Saint and the arms of the Abbey (Argent a cross fleury between four martlets sable) emblazoned on the folio containing the Proemium. The Calendar contains an entry "Dedication of the Church of Abingdon" under the date 10 Kal. Nov: (23 Oct.). The MS. was later owned by Dr Richard Bartlet. Other names, apparently of owners, which appear in it are John Baticumbe and Richardus Lofthous. It was at one period lent by Dr Clayton to Brian Twyne,[1] who made some notes in it.[2]

(2) *Harley MS. No. 3 in the British Museum.*

A late fourteenth-century MS. of 304 folios, containing only the text without the additional matter found in the Pembroke College copy. It was purchased by Dr John Dee from the widow of Mr Carye on the 3rd of August 1573. It afterwards belonged to Sir Simon d'Ewes, and finally entered the Harleian collection which was later transferred to the British Museum.

(3) *Lambeth Palace Library MS. No. 444, f. 180.*

A fifteenth-century tract bound up with several other MSS. to form one book, which belonged to Archbishop Sancroft. It consists only of the treatise on the "Signs of Death" with the rubric, which we have printed, from which it is evident that the scribe must have known both the *Breviarium* and *Florarium*

---

[1] See Brian Twyne MSS. No. II, f. 96b and No. XXII, f. 374, both in Oxford University Archives.
[2] See Introduction, p. 20.

Bartholomei, but that he confused them. The text is hopelessly corrupt, and there are several gaps in the earlier section covered by the two *Breviarium* MSS., but it contains additional matter at the end.

Sloane MS. 3149, f. 19 and Add. MS. 27582, f. 255, both in the British Museum; and Bodleian MSS. Digby 29, f. 153; Digby 31, f. 73; and Bodley 58, f. 129, are merely fifteenth-century extracts of the opening of Part xv only (which is really based on Bernardus de Gordonio, *De Conservatione Vite Humane*).

In addition to the Plates of the *Breviarium,* which are given in this work, three further Photographs of other folios, including the beginning of the Proemium, will be found in Sir Norman Moore's *History of the Study of Medicine in the British Isles.*

APPENDIX B

NOTES ON THE MSS. OF THE *FLORARIUM BARTHOLOMEI* USED IN THE PREPARATION OF THE TEXT

Considerable difficulty has been experienced in preparing the text of the extracts from the *Florarium Bartholomei* now printed owing to the fact that no thoroughly reliable copy of the work is extant. Sir Norman Moore was of the opinion that Royal MS. 7. F. XI in the British Museum might be in Mirfeld's own handwriting:[1] this theory is, however, untenable, for the manuscript in question is by no means the earliest or most perfect copy of the work. Research has brought to light the several manuscripts which are about to be described, but even now it is not possible to be absolutely certain that the text as presented is that originally penned by John Mirfeld himself; and particularly is this the case, when one is faced with his misquotations from standard books.

Mirfeld's original manuscript of the *Florarium* having been lost, the copies of it which still exist are the work of professional transcribers. At a very early date, perhaps even during the compiler's lifetime, errors of transcription must have crept into the copies that were made, and from these erroneous models two definite series of texts emerge. The better of these is that represented by Gray's Inn MS. No. 4, whilst the more corrupt version appears in the later Royal MS. 7. F. XI. In many places, however, both versions agree in an erroneous reading, and it is also obvious, from an examination of the MSS. themselves, that the transcribers of both versions were puzzled as to the reading of identical words or passages, a fact which makes it highly probable that Mirfeld's original manuscript was not a model of clarity or correctness.

Of the complete work of the *Florarium* only two manuscripts are extant, viz. MS. No. 4 in the possession of the Honourable Society of Gray's Inn, and Royal MS. 7. F. XI now in the British Museum. A copy lacking the opening and closing chapters is MS. Mm. II. IO in the University Library at Cambridge: whilst a complete transcript of the chapter "De Medicis" followed by extracts from some of the opening chapters appears in Sloane MS. No. 59 (at f. 190) in the British Museum. These

---

[1] *Op. cit.* p. 45.

four MSS. all give the chapter "De Medicis" in full, whilst the first two cited contain also the full Prologue and Epilogue.

A manuscript in the library of Sion College, London,[1] viz. MS. Arc. L 40. 2/L. 15, numbered 16 or 4080 in E. Bernard's *Catalogi Librorum Manuscriptorum Angliae et Hiberniae* (Oxford, 1697), is an abridgement of the whole work: whilst Harley MS. No. 106, f. 129, in the British Museum, contains notes of some of the earlier chapters, including that on Physicians. These two MSS. have proved useful adjuncts to the four preceding ones in the formation of the text. All six (which we have labelled A—F) appear more fully described below.

Extracts consisting of one or more chapters of the *Florarium* (but *not* of the chapter "De Medicis") are found in MSS. Dd. xi. 83, f. 64b, in Cambridge University Library; in St John's College, Cambridge, MS. No. 125; Corpus Christi College, Oxford, MS. No. ccxxvi, f. 135 in Coxe's Catalogue (under the name "Bartholomeus Anglicus"); and Magdalen College, Oxford, MS. No. lxxii, f. 142b (Coxe). Balliol College MS. No. lxxxviii (Coxe) appeared at first sight to be a copy of the *Florarium*, but a closer examination proved that this was not the case.

It would appear from the notebook compiled by John Bale (Bishop of Ossory) between the years 1549 and 1557[2] that the Library of Oxford University possessed, at that date, a MS. of the *Florarium*: but this copy, which does not appear in the catalogues drawn up in 1439 and 1443, had disappeared before the foundation of the Bodleian in 1603, nor has any trace of it been discovered since.

It would seem, too, from the catalogue compiled between the years 1504–1526 (and now MS. No. 141 in Corpus Christi College, Cambridge[3]) that the Syon Monastery[4] at Isleworth possessed two copies of the *Florarium*, one (I. 27) consisting of excerpts, being catalogued as the *Florarium Bartholomei*, whilst the other (L. 17) is ascribed to Bartholomeus Anglicus (i.e. De Glanville, author of the *De Proprietatibus Rerum*), a writer with whom Mirfeld is sometimes confused, but whom, as a matter of

---

[1] Founded 1630: formerly situated in London Wall, now located on the Victoria Embankment.

[2] Bodleian Library, MS. Selden Supra 64 (Bernard No. 3452), at f. 14 under the heading "Bartholomeus quidam Anglus" ("Ex bibliotheca Academie Oxon."). Edited by R. Lane Poole in *Anecdota Oxoniensia*, Mediaeval and Modern Series, Vol. iv, Part ix (1902) as John Bale's *Index Britanniae Scriptorum* (p. 38). For this point see also H. H. E. Craster in the *Bodleian Quarterly Record*; No. 20, p. 197 and No. 21, p. 207.

[3] Edited by Mary Bateson (Cambridge University Press, 1898).

[4] Dissolved by Henry VIII: it must not be confused with Sion College, London (now the owner of MS. E).

fact, he quotes by name in the *Breviarium*.[1] Of these copies all trace has been lost.

The following MSS., which we have labelled A—F, have been used for the text; they have been arranged, not in order of date of transcription, but in order of merit regarded from the point of view of their value for the text. Gray's Inn MS. No. 4, which we have called A, has been taken as the standard text, but it is by no means perfect, and therefore minor errors have been corrected, and missing words supplied, by reference to the other texts. Where, however, variant readings offer important differences, these have been shown in footnotes; and where all the MSS. agree, but are obviously in error (e.g. the extract from the *Secret of Secrets*, on p. 136), the text has been transcribed as it stands, with a footnote giving the correct version, whilst the error has been disregarded in the translation.

The further details which we now give in regard to the six MSS. used in the preparation of the Text may prove of interest:

MS. A. *Gray's Inn MS. No. 4.*

Referred to as "A" in the footnotes to the Latin text. A MS. copy of the complete work (written in a style of handwriting common at the end of the fourteenth century), containing 333 folios. Nothing is known of its provenance, history, or previous ownership beyond the fact that it was in the possession of the Benchers of the Inn as early as the year 1697 when Bernard's catalogue was published. The text of this MS. has been used as far as possible as the basis of the edition, as its readings generally appear to be the most correct: it is not, however, free from corruptions, and occasionally, too, an hiatus occurs.

MS. B. *British Museum, Royal MS. 7. F. XI.*

Referred to as "B". An early fifteenth-century copy of the complete work, the text of which is hopelessly corrupt. An attempt at correction was made in the fifteenth century, but was soon discontinued. This book once belonged to Thomas Baxter, parson of Stikeford, and afterwards to the Order of the Trinity (or "Bonhommes") of Ashridge in Buckinghamshire, to whom it was given in 1518 by Richard Hutton, as recorded in the following notes which are found after the table of chapters at the end of the text on f. 259: "Iste liber constat

---

[1] The reference is to the *Breviarium*, Part VI (Genitals), Dist. 1, chapter 13 ("Nocturnal Pollution"): "Dicit Bartholomeus in libro suo de proprietatibus rerum quod semen lactuce tam siluestris quam domestice libidinosas ymaginaciones in sompnis compescit".

172   JOHANNES DE MIRFELD

Thome Baxster, vicario perpetuo ecclesie Parochialis de Stik-
ford": (then, lower down, in a different handwriting) "Richardus Hutton: Qui Richardus contulit istum librum domui
religiose de Asherug ibidem in biblioteca permansurum. Anno
domini, 1518." It had found its way into the Royal Library
before the middle of the sixteenth century, for it is obviously
this copy of the *Florarium Bartholomei* which is located "Ex
bibliotheca anglorum regis" according to an entry on f. 193 of
Bishop Bale's notebook.[1] It was ultimately transferred with the
rest of the royal collection to its present home in the British
Museum.

MS. C. *Cambridge University Library, MS. Mm. II. 10 (or No. 2305).*

Referred to in the notes as "C". Described in Luard's catalogue as *Sermones*, or *Loci Communes*, this is actually a fifteenth-
century copy of the *Florarium Bartholomei*,[2] but imperfect, however, at both the beginning and the end. It lacks the Prologue
and the opening twenty-two chapters, and begins with part of the
chapter "De Consuetudine": from this point onwards the manuscript is intact until chapter CLXVIII, "De Veritate", is reached,
but the succeeding chapters and the Epilogue are missing.
Fortunately, the chapter "De Medicis" has survived (at
f. 119b). The MS. as it now exists, in its mutilated state, contains
260 folios written in double columns of 48 lines each. The text
generally follows A, and both MSS. would seem to have been
copied from originals which were illegible or obscure in identical
places. There is no indication as to when, or how, the missing
folios were lost. The book belonged to Sir Thomas Knyvett of
Ashwellthorpe during the earlier part of the seventeenth
century, and then passed into the library of John Moore,
Bishop of Ely 1707–1714; which collection, after the prelate's
death, was purchased in 1715 and presented to the University
of Cambridge by King George I. It was appropriate that
Bishop Moore should have owned a copy of Mirfeld's work,
for during the years 1689–1691 he was Rector of St Andrew's,
Holborn.

MS. D. *British Museum, Sloane MS. 59, f. 190.*

Referred to as "D". This consists of the chapter "De
Medicis" copied out in full, followed immediately (at f. 194b)
by the title written partly in cypher: "Fl4r1r35[m]

[1] Bodleian Library, MS. Selden Supra 64 (No. 3452 in Bernard's catalogue), written *circ.* 1549–1557.
    [2] This identification was made by G. R. Owst in his *Preaching in Medieval
England* (Cambridge, 1926).

Birth4l4m23 Capitulo de medicis et medicinis". Then come short excerpts from the Prologue, and the first forty-four chapters, "Abstinencia–Elemosina". The text is in general agreement with the corrupt version B, but does, however, give some readings from the better text; e.g. "Casteyn" and not "Castym". The *Florarium* excerpt forms one article (No. 11) out of fifteen miscellaneous medical tracts copied out by different scribes and bound up together to form one manuscript of 214 folios, and is written in a late fifteenth-century hand not dissimilar to that of E. According to a note on f. 1 b, this manuscript was once given to Peterhouse, Cambridge, by Dr John Somerset, physician to Henry VI (who also, in 1454, bestowed upon the College a book still in its possession and now numbered MS. 231), a life interest in it being reserved for Roger Marchall, viz. "Egregius arcium medicineque doctor Magister Johannes Somerseth donauit hunc librum medicine Collegio Sancti Petri Cantabrigie cuius tamen vsum habebit M. Rogerus Marchall per totam vitam suam." The subsequent history of the MS. is obscure until its arrival in the Sloane collection.

MS. E. *Sion College MS. Arc. L 40.2/L. 15 (f. 1).*

(No. 16, or No. 4080 in Bernard's catalogue): referred to as "E". A late fifteenth-century abridgment of the whole work, the text being of the same recension as A, containing the Prologue and Epilogue in full, and each chapter, including that on "Physicians", in a very shortened form. Unhappily the folio which contained both the reference to "Casteyn" wine, and also the extract from Bernardus de Gordonio on the nature of the stomach, has been torn out; perhaps to make more easily available the rules of diet which it contained. Nothing is known of the history of this MS. beyond the fact that the book was presented to the College in 1664 by a London clergyman, viz. the Rev. John Bradshaw, Rector of St George, Botolph Lane, and was saved from perishing in the Fire of London. The note following the colophon is dealt with in the Introduction.[1]

Following the abbreviated text of the *Florarium* comes a series of notes, consisting chiefly of Mirfeld's definitions of the subjects that he treats. These are termed "Distinctions of Virtues and Vices", thus exemplifying the fact that the book was regarded as a "speculum".

MS F. *British Museum, Harley MS. 106, f. 129 (Article 70).*

Referred to as "F". This consists of a series of notes from the *Florarium*, taken, apparently at random, from about thirty of the

[1] See p. 102.

first ninety chapters, beginning with the Prologue and extending as far as the chapter "De Monachis". The text followed seems to be that of A. This MS. does not contain any reference to "Casteyn" wine, or to the "parts" of the stomach, but is useful in one or two minor particulars. Thus it has the marginal note "Contra curatos" against "spiritual physicians", for which see the Notes to the Translation (p. 133). This is possibly the earliest of all the MSS., and would seem, from its calligraphy, to have been copied out in Mirfeld's lifetime. For this point, and the remark with which it is prefaced, see the Introduction (p. 99). It is merely one article (No. 70) among one hundred and fifty-six other manuscript tracts bound up together as one book.

Two folios of the British Museum MS. 7 F.XI of the *Florarium*, containing the beginning of the Proemium and of the Chapter "De Medicis" respectively, will be found reproduced in Sir Norman Moore's *History of the Study of Medicine in the British Isles*, to which reference has been made in the Text.

APPENDIX C

ABSTRACTS FROM DEEDS & DOCUMENTS REFERRED TO IN THE TEXT

(arranged for the most part in the order in which
they occur therein)

I

*Extracts from the Ordination Lists contained in the Register of
Richard Braybroke, Bishop of London 1381–1404
(Bishop of London's Registry)*

(a) WILLIAM MIRFELD THE YOUNGER[1]

Saturday, 23 September 1391. William Mirfeld of York diocese
(by letters dimissory from York diocese), Acolyte and Subdeacon: Title, The Hospital of St Bartholomew in Smethefeld,
London.

Saturday, 1 March 1392 [i.e. 1393]. William Mirfeld, perpetual
vicar of the parish church of "Ledes" in the diocese of York,
ordained priest by letters dimissory from York diocese.

(b) JOHANNES DE MIRFELD[2]

Saturday, 19 September 1394. Ordinations in St Paul's Cathedral.
Acolyte: "Johannes Mirfeld, Ciuitatis Londonie, iste non fuit
ordinatus" (this man was not ordained).

Saturday, 6 March 1394 [i.e. 1395]. Ordinations in St Paul's
Cathedral. Acolyte: John Mirfeld, of the diocese of London.
On the same day, John Mirfeld, of the City of London,
Acolyte, was advanced to the order of Subdeacon: Title,
..."Magistri et Confraternitatis hospitalis Sancti Bartholomei
in Smethefeld Londonie".

Saturday, 27 March 1395. In the conventual church of St
Trinity, Aldgate. John Mirfeld, of the City of London, Subdeacon, was ordained Deacon: Title, The Master and Confraternity of the Hospital of St Bartholomew, Smethefeld.

Saturday, 10 April 1395. In St Trinity, Aldgate. John Mirfeld,
of the City of London, ordained Priest: Title, "The Master and
Confraternity of St Bartholomew, Smethefeld 'ciuitatis
eiusdem'".

[1] *Supra* p. 16.   *Supra* pp. 7, 8.

II

Will of John Mirfeld[1]

Register of wills proved in the Court of the Archdeacon of London, Register No. 1 (1393–1415), f. 172 (Principal Probate Registry, Somerset House)

Memorandum quod xvij Kalendas Maij Anno domini Millesimo CCCC^{mo} Septimo Dominus Johannes Meryfeld Capellanus in bona et sana memoria sua existens suum testamentum nuncupatiuum condidit et fecit in hunc modum. In primis legauit animam etc. ac corpus suum ad sepeliendum in cimiterio sancti Botolphi extra Aldrichgate Londonie. Item dedit et legauit Margarete Schadelok matri sue omnia bona sua mobilia et immobilia vbicunque existencia ad persoluenda debita sua et vlterius ad faciendum ordinandum et disponendum de eisdem bonis pro anima sua et animabus omnium fidelium defunctorum prout saluti anime sue proficere melius eis videbitur expedire. Huius autem testamenti sui nuncupatiui fecit et constituit predictam Margaretam executricem suam. Hiis testibus domino Waltero Compton capellano Roberto Peterburgh ac Johanne Stonham. Datum Londonie die et Anno domini supradictis.

Probatum etc. iij Nonas Maij Anno domini supradicto etc. Et commissa est administracio omnium bonorum etc. executrici superius nominate iurate primitus in forma iuris et admissa per eandem.

Translation

Memorandum that on the xvii Kalends of May in the year of Our Lord 1407, Dominus John Meryfeld, Chaplain, being sound in mind and of good understanding, made and composed his nuncupative testament in this form. Firstly, he bequeathed his soul, etc. [i.e. to God, St Mary, and the Saints] and his body to be buried within the cemetery of St Botolph Without Aldersgate in London. Item, he gave and bequeathed to Margaret Schadelok his mother all his property both moveable and immoveable wherever it should be found, for the payment of his debts, and then to be so dealt with, ordered, and disposed of for the good of his soul and the souls of all the faithful departed as it shall seem to them (*sic*) to be most expedient for the good of his soul. And of this his nuncupative testament he made and constituted the aforesaid Margaret his executrix, there being present as witnesses thereunto Dominus Walter Compton, Chaplain, Robert Peterburgh, and John Stonham. Dated at London the day and year of Our Lord above mentioned.

Proved, etc., on the iii Nones of May in the year of Our Lord above mentioned, etc. And the administration of all the goods, etc., was granted to the above-named executrix, and after she had been sworn in due form of law she was admitted by the same.

[1] *Supra* p. 8.

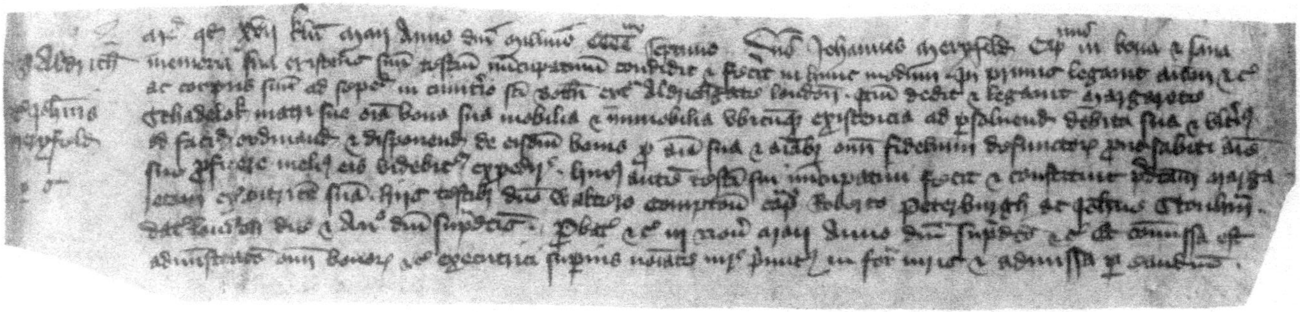

Plate IV

WILL OF JOHANNES DE MIRFELD

Photograph of the entry relating to Johannes de Mirfeld in the Register
of Wills, proved in the Court of the Archdeacon of London, 1393–1415

III

Translation...Hustings Roll No. 107; Deed No. 135
(preserved in the Guildhall of the City of London)[1]

KNOW ALL MEN present and future that I John Mirfeld have
given, granted, and by this my present charter have confirmed,
to John Herthull, clerk, all those tenements with the houses, and
shops built thereon, gates, walls, gardens, etc. and all other the
appurtenances thereof, which lately came to me and to William
atte Vyne, citizen of London, on the deaths of Dom. William
de Mirfeld and of Dom. Roger de Barnesborgh, clerks, by grant
from Elias de Sutton, clerk; situated in the parish of St Andrew
de Holbourne, in the suburb of London (the said William atte
Vyne having, for himself and his heirs for ever, by charter
dated before these presents, released and quitted-claim to me the
aforesaid John and to my heirs for ever, all the right which he
had, could have, or ever shall have, to all the aforesaid tenements
with the appurtenances thereof as aforesaid): To HAVE AND TO
HOLD to the aforesaid John Herthull during the whole term of
his life of the capital lord of that fee for the services thence due
and of right accustomed; and after the death of the said John
Herthull, all the aforesaid tenements...are to remain fully
over to Master Adam Rous, surgeon to the Lord King of
England and his heirs and assigns to have and to hold to the
said Adam Rous... for ever. I HAVE ALSO GIVEN... to the
said John Herthull all those tenements, etc., of which I, the said
John Mirfeld, William atte Vyne, and Robert Bryen, received
joint possession lately by the gift and feoffment of the aforesaid
Master Adam in the parishes of "St Mildrithe in Pulletria" (in
the Poultry) London, and in St Edmund the King in "Lum-
bardestret", and in "Bercherneslane", London, and of which
the said William and Robert have already quitted-claim to
me...: TO HOLD to John Herthull for life and then to remain
over to the said Master Adam to have and to hold ... to him
for ever... [Warranty to John Herthull for life, and then to
the heirs of Adam Rous]. Witnesses, Simon Wynchecombe,
John Bewfrount, John Brounesbury, butcher, Roger Legat,
John Totenale. Dated, London, 1st April, 2 Richard II [1379].

Enrolled on Monday after the feast of St John before the
Latin Gate, 2 Richard II [9 May 1379].

[1] *Supra* p. 9.

IV

Abstracts of deeds, dated 47 Edward III [1373], from Hustings Roll No. 102 (preserved in the Guildhall of the City of London)[1]

The following deeds were all enrolled together on the Monday next after the feast of St Katherine the Virgin, 48 Edward III (i.e. 27 November 1374).

(1) *Deed No. 178:*

Quit-claim by Roger de Barneburgh, clerk, to Dom. Elias de Sutton, clerk, of the messuage or inn formerly belonging to John Tavy in St Andrew's, Holborn, on the south side of the highway: AND ALSO of that formerly belonging to Sir W. de Newenham which Barneburgh and Sutton obtained jointly [in 1366 and 1363 respectively]: Dated, London 14 July, 47 Edw. III [1373]. Witnesses, Stephen de Holbourn, Roger Legat, Henry Godechep, John de Totenhale, Roger de Podyngton, Hugh le Clerc.

(2) *Deed No. 179:*

Grant by William de Mirfeld, clerk, to Dom. Elias de Sutton, clerk, of the tenements, etc., he had by the feoffment [in 1370] of Nigel West (executor of Dom. Thomas de Cotyngham) in St Andrew's, Holborn. Dated, 18 July 1373. Witnesses as above.

(3) *Deed No. 180:*

Grant by Elias de Sutton, clerk, to Dom. William de Mirfeld, clerk, and Roger de Barneburgh, clerk, for their lives, with remainder to John de Mirfeld and William atte Vyne, citizen of London, of his tenements [i.e. "Newenham's"] situated between those formerly of Dom. Thomas de Cotyngham on the east and Stephen de Holbourn on the west; extending in length from that of John de Tamworth on the south to the highway at a point opposite to the house of the Bishop of Ely in Holbourn on the north, in the suburb of London. Dated, 23 July 1373. Witnesses as above.

(4) *Deed No. 181:*

Grant by Elias de Sutton, clerk, to Dom. William de Mirfeld, clerk, for life, with remainder to John de Mirfeld and William atte Vyne, citizen of London, of all his tenement, etc. [i.e. "Tavy's"], in St Andrew's, Holborn, situated between the tenement of the Master and Brethren of the Hospital of St Bartholomew de Smethefeld in which Sir John Moubray, knight, lately dwelt, on the west; the house in which Hugh le Clerc now

[1] *Supra* p. 13.

lives on the east; the highway of Holbourn on the north; and the garden of William de Norton on the south: AND ALSO of his other tenement [i.e. "Cotyngham's"] situated between the tenement formerly of Sir William de Newenham on the west, that of the Hospital on the east, and which extends in length from the highway on the north to the tenement of the Hospital on the south. Dated, London, 23 July 1373.

Thus on the 23rd of July 1373 the ownership of the series of properties on the south side of Holborn from east to west was vested in the following:

(1) Hugh le Clerc.
(2) William de Mirfeld (formerly Tavy), remainder to John de Mirfeld and William atte Vyne.
(3) St Bartholomew's Hospital.
(4) William de Mirfeld (formerly Cotyngham), remainder to John de Mirfeld and William atte Vyne.
(5) William de Mirfeld and Roger de Barnesburgh jointly (formerly Newenham), remainder to John de Mirfeld and William atte Vyne.
(6) Stephen de Holbourn.

V

William de Mirfeld the Elder

Chancery Inquisitiones Post Mortem, Edward III
(Public Record Office, London)[1]

Inquisitio Post Mortem held at Normanton, co. York, the 30th of December, 49 Edward III (1375).

William de Mirfeld, clerk, held in chief on the day of his death the manors of Fersley and Shelff in co. York, by service of one penny per annum. Joan de Mirfeld, one of his sisters, and John de Mirfeld, son of Margaret de Mirfeld his other sister, are his next heirs, and are of full age, both being upwards of forty years or more. He died 25 July last.

(The jury included John de Fourneys, Adam de Dodworth, and William Shelyto.)

[As a result of the findings of this inquisition, the Escheator for Yorkshire was, on the 26th of January 1376, ordered to take the fealties of Joan and John Mirfeld and to divide the manors equally between them. (*Calendar of Fine Rolls*, Vol. VIII (1368–1377), p. 337.) Evidently Joan took Shelf and John received Fersley.]

[1] *Supra* p. 14.

VI

Will of William de Mirfeld the Elder[1]

Archdeaconry of London Wills, Register No. 1 (Principal Probate Registry, Somerset House)

In the Index of wills proved before the Official (the originals and registered copies of which are lost) under the year 1375 occurs the following entry:

"Test[amentum] Will[ielm]i de Mirfeld canonici Lincoln-[ensis] ff. xlvj."

(The entry "Canon of Lincoln" seems to have been added later.)

William died, as we have seen (p. 179), on July 25, 1375).

VII

On 23 January 1374, William de Mirfeld, the King's Clerk, and parson of the church of Bradford[1], obtained (for 6s. 8d.) the royal licence to alienate in mortmain to William de Cotes, vicar of the said church, a messuage in Bradford as a habitation for himself and his successors. (*Calendar of Patent Rolls*, 1370–1374, p. 387.)

On 15 July 1375, William de Mirfeld, clerk, and Roger de Barneburgh, clerk, obtained a royal licence to alienate certain lands in mortmain to Kirklees Nunnery [traditional scene of Robin Hood's death]. (*Calendar of Patent Rolls*, 1374–1377, p. 126.)

VIII

Abstracts from "Feet of Fines for the County of York, 1347–1377" (printed in Yorkshire Archaeological Society Record Series, Vol. LII (1914))[2]

Page 67 [No. 39]. Quindene of Michaelmas, 32 Edward III, 1358. Final concord by which William de Mirfeld [afterwards Sir William de Mirfeld] in return for 100 marks obtains from Adam de Helay of Mirfeld the acknowledgment of his right to 4s. rent and one-fourth part of 200 acres of pasture and 200 acres of moor in Mirfeld, together with the homage and service of Adam de Hopton, Thomas de Essholf, Hugh Pykard, chaplain, William de Mirfeld, clerk, Richard de Northorp, John Sumpter, and their heirs.

[According to Dodsworth MS. No. 117, f. 149 (Bodleian Library) Adam de Heley granted his interest in a fourth part of

---

[1] *Supra* p. 12.   [2] *Supra* p. 11, note 2.

the seignory of Mirfield to William Mirfield, in 23 Edward III.]

Page 145 [No. 10]. Quindene of Easter, 44 Edward III, 1370. William de Fyncheden, chivaler, William de Mirfeld, parson of the church of Bradford, William de Mirfeld, "chivaler", and others, are associated together as demandants (i.e. plaintiffs) in a fine.

[Sir William de Mirfeld, knight, Conservator of the Peace for co. York, was a man of considerable importance in the West Riding, and was head of the Mirfield family. His association with the elder William de Mirfeld the priest in this fine is proof that the two men were relatives, otherwise he would not have permitted the Chancery Clerk to use the name of Mirfeld.]

Page 145 [No. 7]. Quindene of Hilary, 44 Edward III, 1370. William de Mirfeld, Roger de Barneburgh, and Elias de Sutton, clerks, are the three demandants in a fine of lands in Campsall and Burghwallis near Doncaster.

IX

Extracts from the will of Roger de Barneburgh proved in the London Commissary Court (Bishop Courtenay's Register, f. 18b), Principal Probate Registry, Somerset House[1]

Roger de Barneburgh, clerk, Canon of All Saints, Derby.... If he shall happen to die in London, then he is to be buried in the chapel of St Katherine in St Bartholomew's, Smithfield; and in that case leaves twenty marks to the Prior and Convent on condition that they "make a special mention" on behalf of his soul in the Masses to be celebrated for Dom. William de Merfeld. Bequests to the altar, etc., of St Andrew's, Holborn.

A legacy to his kinswoman Margaret wife of William de Dodworth. Bequeaths to John de Conwyk a bowl with a cover to it "which Dom. William de Merifyld left me".

To Adam de Miryfild, tailor, ten marks.

Mentions also certain money which he is bound to distribute on behalf of William de Mirfeld in the parishes of "Mekesbrugh" [i.e. Mexborough], Strensall, and Nassington.

Leaves to Elias de Sutton all the black cloths which he provided for the funeral of William de Mirfeld.

Executors, Elias de Sutton, John de Conewyk de Herthull, and others.

Dated, London, 4 August 1375. Proved 17 Kalend. Nov. (16 October) following.

[1] *Supra* pp. 12, 16.

X

Inquisitio Post Mortem held on the Saturday next after Michaelmas, 1 Richard II. [3 Oct. 1377.][1]

John son of John de Fourneys de Mirfeld held in chief on the day of his death the manor of Ferslay and eight bovates of land in Ferslay valued at 40 shillings per annum. He died on Thursday next before the Decollation of St John Baptist last past [i.e. 27 August].

His heir is his brother Adam de Fourneys de Mirfeld, who is aged forty years or more.

Inquisitio Post Mortem held 7 March, 4 Richard II [1381][2].

Joan Mirfeld, sister of William de Mirfeld clerk, held part of the manor of Shelf. She died on 22 December last. Her heirs are her daughters, viz. Beatrice, wife of John de Morhous, and aged fifty years or more; Sibyl, wife of William Shillyto, aged forty years; Margaret, wife of Adam de Dodeworth, aged thirty years; and Cecily, wife of John Fustour, aged thirty-six years.

Extract from the Calendar of Patent Rolls, 1381–1385, p. 187[1].

12 November 1382. Licence (obtained for 40s. by Robert de Swyllyngton, Knight) for Adam Fourneys of Mirfeld, goldsmith of London, to enfeoff the said Robert (and others) of his manor of Ferslay, co. York, held in chief.

Extract from the Calendar of Close Rolls, 1381–1385, p. 223[1].

Grant by Adam Fourneys de Mirfeld, goldsmith of London, to Robert de Swillyngton, Knight, Thomas de Thornour and Margaret his wife (heirs and assigns of the said Robert) of the manor of Fersley, formerly belonging to William de Mirfled (*sic*) clerk. Dated at Westminster, 14 November, 6 Richard II, 1382; and acknowledged on 24 November.

XI

Extracts from two other wills of members of the Mirfeld family in London[3]

2 January 1394. Adam Mirifeld citizen and goldsmith of London. To be buried in the cemetery of St Paul's called "Pardonchirchehawe" by the side of Agnes his late wife. Bequests to Matilda his present wife, his son Thomas, and his daughter Joan.

(London Commissary Court Wills, Register of Courtney, f. 330; Principal Probate Registry, Somerset House.)

[1] *Supra* p. 15.   [2] *Supra* pp. 14, 15.   [3] *Supra* pp. 15, 16.

5 September 1407. Thomas Mirifeld goldsmith of London. To be buried where his father is. Bequests of gowns to his kinsman Nicholas Mirfeld, and to Adam, brother of the said Nicholas. Leaves a gown to his "bastard brother" John Mannyng. Bequests to his sister Joan and to his mother Matilda (who is named executrix).

(Archdeaconry of London Wills, Register No. 1, f. 104; Principal Probate Registry, Somerset House.)

[According to a writ of supersedeas issued 19 June 1388, Nicholas Mirfelde and Adam Mirfelde, "taillour" of London, stood bail together for Richard Wellis. (*Calendar of Close Rolls,* 1385–1389, p. 496.)]

XII

Extract from the *Calendar of Close Rolls, 1377–1381, p. 247*[1].

Indenture between Sir Robert de Swyllyngton and Master Adam Rous of the Poultry, surgeon in the City of London, witnessing the grant (at a rent) to Adam and his heirs of land, etc., in Normanton and Sutton upon Sore co. Nottingham. Dated and acknowledged, 20 May, 2 Richard II, 1379.

[William de Mirfeld the Younger exchanged the living of Leeds for that of Swillington (the patronage of which belonged to the family of Sir Robert de Swillington) by royal licence dated 8 August 1393. (*Calendar of Patent Rolls,* 1391–1396, p. 310.)]

[1] *Supra* p. 15.

INDEX

Abingdon Abbey, 167
Acrostics in (a) *Breviarium*, 39–41;
   (b) *Florarium*, 99, 100
Afflacius, Johannes, 69
Alexander the Great, 111, 137
Amber, use of, as a medicine, 89
Ambrose, St (Archbishop of Milan), 159
Apothecaries' weight, 93
Appendices, 166–183
   A. MSS. used for the text of the
      Breviarium, 167, 168
   B. MSS. used for the text of the
      Florarium, 169–174
   C. Abstracts from Deeds and
      Documents referred to in the
      text, 175–183
Aquinas, St Thomas, 134
Arabian Medicine, 25–28
Archimatthaeus the Salernitan, 105, 125
Arderne, John of, 105, 123, 132
Aretaeus, 65, 69
Aristotle, 28, 31, 51, 111, 112, 137
Arnold of Villanova, 30
Artemisia (mugwort), use of, in
   prognosis, 67
Asa, King of Judah, 159
Avicenna, 28, 44, 79, 143, 157
   — the *Canon*, 28, 43, 50, 62, 77, 83, 84
   — the *Cantica*, 153
Avoirdupois weight, 93

Banana, *see* Musa
Barley-water, 81
Barnesburgh, Roger de, 9, 10, 12–14,
   16, 177–179, 181
Bartholomaeus Anglicus, 170, 171
Bartholomaeus Florarius, 99
Bartholomaeus of Salerno, 30, 43, 75
Bartlet, Dr Richard, 167
Bartlett's Buildings, Holborn, 14
Baths, for consumptives, 87
   — relation of food to, 155
Bede, the Venerable, 119, 127, 159
Bernard Sylvester (of Chartres), 130

Bernardus de Gordonio, 28, 31
— — *De Conservatione Vite Humane*,
   113, 135, 139, 141, 146, 147,
   149–155, 173
— — *De Decem Ingeniis Curandorum
   Morborum*, 122, 133
— — *Lilium Medicine*, 43, 77–79,
   113, 143, 149, 151
Bile, 32, 61, 69
Bleeding, *see* Phlebotomy
Blood, 32, 61, 69
— an examination of, an aid in
   prognosis, 69
"Bolus armeniacus" (an astringent
   medicine), 89
Book of the Foundation of St Bartholo-
   mew's, 2
Braybroke, Robert de (Bishop of
   London), Register of, 4, 7, 16,
   175
Breviarium Bartholomei, 36–95
— — Acrostic in, 39–41
— — Authority, based on, 41–44,
   95
— — Authorship, proof of, 39, 40
— — Charms in, 43, 44, 67–71
— — Complete text of, 37
— — Composition, date of, 7, 25,
   38
— — Construction and contents
   of, 41–45
— — Consumption, *see* Phthisis
— — *De Signis Malis*, chapter on,
   43, 45, 54–73, 167
— — "Emplastrum Bartholomei",
   45, 90, 91
— — Epilogue, 45, 94, 95
— — Gunpowder, directions for
   making, 45, 90, 91
— — Introductory Remarks to,
   36–45
— — Magic and superstition in,
   43, 44, 67–71
— — MSS. sources of, 37, 167, 168
— — Nature of the work, 36, 41,
   105

Breviarium Bartholomei, Phthisis (Ptisis), chapter on, 43–45, 74–89; *see also special entry* Phthisis
— — Prayer for use when preparing and taking medicine, 40, 41, 44, 71
— — *Proemium* (Preface) to, 45–53
— — "Quid pro Quo", 37, 167
— — Reasons for writing the Book, 36, 47–51, 101
— — Rubrics, explanatory in, 39–41
— — "Signs of Death", *see* "De Signis Malis"
— — *Sinonoma Bartholomei* (Glossary), *see special entry*
— — Size of, voluminous, viii, 41
— — "Weights and Measures", extract on, 45, 92, 93
British Museum, notes on MSS. of Johannes de Mirfeld's works at, 167–174
Bromyard, John, 99, 103
Bruno of Calabria, 122

Calendar, astronomical, of John Somer, 22, 38, 167
— — of Walter de Elvesden, 37
Candle of herbs, use of, in medicine, 67–69
Canon Law, 106–111, 127–131, 134, 139
Capsula Eburnea, 27, 62–65, 71
Carphology, 59, 73
Casteyn (Chestnut) wine from Provence, 148, 149, 173, 174
Castoreum, 85
Charms, the use of, 43, 44, 67–71, 123
Chartularies of the Priory and Hospital of St Bartholomew, 16
Chaucer, 3, 31, 107, 132
Cheese, as food, 145–147
Chishull, John (capellanus), 17–19
Church, medieval, attitude of, towards medicine, 107–111
Cinquefoil, its use in prognosis, 71
Complexion, the, 32, 155
Conduct, professional, 125–127
Constantinus Africanus, 27–29, 47, 50, 69, 157
Consumption, *see* Phthisis

"Contra curatos" ("Spiritual Physicians", Parish Priests), 104, 133–135, 174
"Contra feminas qui se intromittunt de Phisica", 122, 123
Contraceptives, 44
Council, of Rheims (A.D. 1131), 109
— the Fourth Lateran (A.D. 1215), 110, 128
Crab, *see* River-Crab
"Curatos, contra", *see* "Contra curatos"

De Medicis et Eorum Medicinis, chapter from the *Florarium* on, 122–159
— — — Cheese as a food, 145–147
— — — Church, the medieval, in relation to medicine, 107–111
— — — Diet, advice on, 136, 137, 143–157
— — — Digestion, medieval theory of, 149–153
— — — Exercise, value and varieties of, 137–143
— — — "Irregularity", danger of incurring, 129–131
— — — Physicians, education of, 110, 123; fees of, 127, 131–135; indictment of, 49, 106, 107, 131–133; professional conduct, advice in regard to, 105–107, 125, 126; qualifications and duties of, 123–131; *see also special entry* Physicians
— — — Preservation of Health, advice on, 111–113, 136–157
— — — Spiritual needs of Patients first require attention, 108, 127
— — — Stomach, anatomy of, 151
— — — Wine, good for all complexions, 147–149
— — — Women doctors, 122, 123
De Signis Malis, "the Signs of Death", 43, 45, 54–73, 167
Diarrhoea in Phthisis, treatment of, 87–89
Diet, for consumptives, 81–85
— general advice and directions on, 135–137, 143–157
"Digestio" of fever, 51, 60, 61
Digestion, medieval theory of, 31, 32, 149–153

Dog, the, a medium for prognosis, 67
Dragon's-blood, *see* "Sanguis draconis"

Edward III, 112; his surgeon, Adam Rous, *see* Rous, Adam
Edward, the Black Prince, xi, 3, 45
Electuary for consumptives, 85
"Elements", the four, 32
Elvesden, Walter de, astronomical calendar of, 37
"Emplastrum Bartholomei", 45, 90, 91
Emprosthotonos, of tetanus, 65, 69
Epilogue of (*a*) *Breviarium*, 45, 94, 95; (*b*) *Florarium*, 45, 98, 160–163
Exercise, advice on, 137–143
Exorcism, 108, 109
Experimenter, the (Rhazes), 67
Experiments (unorthodox or untried remedies), use of, 50, 51
Extreme Unction, 108

Fees, medical, 73, 111, 127, 131–135
Fitz-Stephen, 143
Flesh, as food in Phthisis, 81–85
Florarium Bartholomei (the Flower-garden of Bartholomew), 45, 98–163, 169–174
—— Acrostic in, 99, 100
—— Authority, based on, 104, 105, 111–113, 119
—— Composition, date of, 25, 102, 103
—— Construction of, 98
—— *De Medicis et Eorum Medicinis*, chapter on, 122–159; *see also* special entry
—— Dedication to John de Suthwelle, 99, 101, 115
—— Epilogue, 160–163
—— "Flower-garden of Bartholomew", the, 117
—— Headings of chapters in, 164
—— Introductory Remarks to, 98–113
—— MSS. sources of, 98, 169–174
—— Nature of the work, 103–105
—— *Proemium* (Preface) to, 114–121
—— Proof of authorship, 99, 100
—— Reasons for writing, 101, 103, 115–121

Florarium Bartholomei, "Speculum", an example of, 54, 55, 103, 117
"Flower-garden of Bartholomew", the, 117
Fulgentius, St, 139

Gaddesden, John of, 21, 87
Galen, Claudius, 26, 27, 42, 44, 133, 137, 143, 147
—— *Methodus Medendi*, 77, 157
Gargle, for consumptives, 85
Gaunt, John of (Duke of Lancaster), 11, 24
Gehazi, 135
George I, 172
Gerard of Cremona, 28, 47, 55, 63
Gilbertus Anglicus, 44
Gluttony, the danger of, 157
Gray's Inn, MS. no. 4, of the *Florarium*, 98, 169, 171
Gunpowder, directions for making, 45, 90, 91

Hali Abbas, 27, 28, 105, 122, 123
Henbane, use of, in prognosis, 69
Herthull, John (clerk), 9, 10, 13, 14, 177
Hippocrates, 26, 42, 77
— *Aphorisms*, 51, 58, 61, 69, 74, 75, 79, 81, 89
— *Prognostics*, 43, 55, 57, 59, 69, 73
— *Regimen in Acute Diseases*, 80, 81
— *Secrets of*, 43, 70, 71
"Hippocratic face", 43, 55
"Hippocratic oath", 105
Holcroft, Richard, 99
Holkham, *Secretum Secretorum* at, 112
Honain ben Isaac, 27, 55, 63
Honey, beneficial for consumptives, 81
— ingredient of Electuary, 85
Honorius III, Pope, 110
Horwood, A. J., Catalogue of MSS. at Gray's Inn, 99, 100
Humbertus de Romanis, 106
Humoral pathology, 31–33
Humours, the doctrine of, 31–33, 155
Hydromel (honey-water), 81
Hypocistis, use of, as medicine, 88

Idiota, medieval example of, 122, 123

Innocent IV, Pope, 129, 130
Inspeximus (Royal), A.D. 1390, of
    Johannes de Mirfeld's Inden-
    ture with the Priory of A.D. 1362,
    5, 6
Iris, the White, aqueous extract of,
    useful in Phthisis, 85
"Irregular", to become, 7, 109,
    129–131
Isaac Judaeus (Isaac ben Solomon),
    28, 144, 145

Jaundice, prognostic indications of,
    61
Jerome, St, 49, 119, 147
Johannes Hispaliensis (John of
    Toledo), 112
John of Milan, 30
John XXI, Pope (Petrus Hispanus),
    110

Ladanum, 67
Lambeth Palace MS. of "De Signis
    Malis", "the Signs of Death",
    43, 54, 167
Lanfranc of Milan, 23, 76, 132, 133
Lateran Council, the Fourth, 110, 128
Leeds, the living of, 16, 175, 183
Leland, John, 20, 99
Lips, lividity of, an ominous sign, 65

Magic and superstition in Mirfeld's
    works, 43, 44, 67–71
Marcellus Empiricus, 49
Marfeldus, see Mirfeld
"Master, My", 10, 22, 23, 43, 76,
    77
Materia peccans, 50
Medicinal treatment of Phthisis,
    85–89
Medicine, clerks in Higher Orders
    forbidden to practise Medicine
    or Surgery, 110, 129
Medieval Medicine, 25–28
Meryfeld, see Mirfeld
Mesue, 51
Milk, Directions for taking, 81, 89,
    145
— Indications for boiling or heat-
    ing before use, 81, 89
— Of value in Phthisis, 81
— Use of, in prognosis, 67, 69

Mirfeld (alternative spellings of
    name: Marfeldus, 99; Mery-
    feld, 3, 176; Mirfelde, 99, 183;
    Mirfield, vii; Mirfield, 11, 182,
    183; Miryfild, 16, 181; Muryfeld,
    17; Myrfeld, 11)
— A Yorkshire family, 11
— Adam de Fourneys de, 15, 182
— Joan de, 14, 15, 179, 182
— Johannes de:
— — As medical writer, 25–34
— — Burial, 8
— — Capellanus (chaplain), 4, 8;
    possibly in Hospital of St Bar-
    tholomew, 24, 25
— — Clerk of the Priory, 3
— — Commorans (sojourner) in
    the Priory of St Bartholomew,
    5, 6
— — Conveyances of property to
    the Priory, 6, 13, 14, 18, 19
— — Death (A.D. 1407), 8
— — From Yorkshire, 16, 24
— — His mother (Margaret Scha-
    delok), 4, 8, 17, 176
— — Indenture with Priory, 5, 6
— — Legal transactions of, 9, 10,
    13–20, 177–179
— — Life of, 3–25
— — Lived in the Priory, 5, 25
— — Medical knowledge derived
    from books, 22–24
— — "My Master", 10, 22, 23,
    43, 76, 77
— — "Never a pupil", 22, 24, 47,
    76
— — Not an Augustinian Canon,
    3–5, 8, 25
— — Not educated at Oxford,
    20–22
— — Ordination, records of, 4, 7,
    8, 175
— — Relationship to William de
    Mirfeld (the elder), 16, 17
— — Trustee for William de Mir-
    feld and others in favour of the
    Priory, 6, 9, 10, 14, 18, 19
— — Will of, 8, 176
— — See also under Breviarium Bar-
    tholomei, De Medicis et Eorum
    Medicinis, Florarium Bartho-
    lomei and Phthisis

Mirfeld, John, son of John de Fourneys de and of Margaret Mirfeld, 15, 179, 182
— Margaret de, 15, 179
— Nicholas, 16, 183
— (Mirifeld), Thomas de, 15, 183
— Sir William de (Kt), 11, 180, 181
— *William de (the elder)*:
— — Bradford, Yorkshire, incumbent of, 12, 180, 181
— — Burial of, 12
— — Chief Attorney to John of Gaunt, 11
— — Commissioner for custody of Great Seal, 12
— — Death in A.D. 1375, 12, 179, 180
— — From Mirfield in Yorkshire, 11
— — "Great Clerk", 11
— — Inquisitio Post Mortem upon, 179
— — King's Clerk in Royal Chancery, 11
— — Property, belonging to, and disposition of, 13–15, 19, 177–179, 182; left in trust for Priory of St Bartholomew, 19
— — Receiver of Petitions in Parliament, 11
— — Relationship to Johannes de Mirfeld, 16, 17
— — Stoke by Nayland, Suffolk, presented to living of, 11
— — Stow in Lindsey, Lincoln, Prebend of, 12
— — Will, 12, 180
— *William de (the younger)*:
— — Chancery Clerk, 16
— — Incumbent, of Leeds, Yorkshire, 16, 175, 183; of Swillington, 16, 183
— — Ordination, dates of, 16, 175; title for, the Hospital of St Bartholomew, 16, 175
Mirfelde, *see* Mirfeld
Mirifeld, *see* Mirfeld
Miryfild, *see* Mirfeld
Miryfild, Adam de, 16, 181
Montpellier, University of, 30, 113
Moore, Sir Norman, 2, 5, 22, 23, 37, 39, 40, 44, 100, 113, 168, 169, 174
Mowat, J. L. G., 2, 4, 37, 167

MSS., used in preparing text of
    (a) *Breviarium*, 37, 166–168;
    (b) *Florarium*, 98, 166, 169–174
Mugwort, *see* Artemisia
Muryfeld, *see* Mirfeld
Musa, use of, in Phthisis, 85
— Aenea, a compound sedative medicine, 67
"My Master", 10, 22, 23, 43, 76, 77
Myrfeld, *see* Mirfeld

Nails, Incurving of, 79
— Lividity of, a grave sign, 59–61, 65
Natural heat, 33
Nettle, use of, in prognosis, 67
Nicolaus Salernitanus, 37

Ointments for consumptives, 86, 87
Onion, as test of death, 69
Ordination Lists, in Register of Bishop Braybroke, 7, 16, 175
Ovid, 119
Oxford, Johannes de Mirfeld not educated at, 20–22
— Meridian of, astronomical calendars based on, 37, 38, 167
— Nicholas Tyngewich, reference to lecture as Professor of Medicine at, 21–22

Parish priests, indictment of ("contra curatos"), 104, 133–135, 174
Pembroke College, Oxford, MS. of *Breviarium*, 22, 37–41, 167
Peter of Blois, 119, 131
Peterhouse, Cambridge, MS. of *Florarium* formerly owned by, 172, 173
Petrus Hispanus (Pope John XXI), 110
Philosopher, the (Aristotle), 51
Phlebotomy, 53, 69, 141, 143
Phlegm (one of the four humours), 32, 33; *see also* Sputum
Phthisis, Chapter from the *Breviarium* on, 43–45, 74–89
— Definition of, 75
— Diagnosis of, 75–77
— Prognosis in, 75, 77–79
— Signs of approaching death in, 79
— Sudden death in, 77

Phthisis, Treatment of, 79–89; with balneotherapy, 87; with barley-water, 81; with diet, 81 ,83–85; with electuary, 85; with gargle, 85; with honey, 81; with hydromel, 81; with milk, 81; with ointments, 87; with pills, 85; with river-crab, 83; with sugar of roses, 83; with wine, 81

Physicians, Education of, 123
— Fees of, 73, 111, 127, 131–135
— Honour due to, 123
— Indictment of, 49, 131–135
— Professional conduct of, advice in regard to, 105–107, 125, 126
— Qualifications and duties of, 123–131
— "Spiritual", *see* "Contra curatos"

Pills, for consumptives, 85
Pits, John, 20, 99
Plagiarism, in medieval writings, 42
"Plaster of Bartholomew", 45, 90, 91
Platearius, Johannes, 23, 30, 43, 75, 76, 78
Pneumoliths, expectoration of, 79
Prayer for use when preparing and taking medicine, 40, 41, 44, 71
Preface, *see* Proemium
Proemium (Preface) of (*a*) *Breviarium*, 45, 46–53, 61; (*b*) *Florarium*, 45, 114–121
Pupil, Johannes de Mirfeld never occupied position of, 22, 24, 47, 76
Puppies (blind), baths for consumptives prepared from, 87
Pythagoras, sphere of, 70, 71

"Quid pro Quo", the, 37, 167

Register of Bishop Braybroke, 7, 16, 175
Rhazes, 28, 43, 62, 67
Richard II, 3, 38
Riley, H. T., 39, 122, 123
River-crab, as food, 83; for preparing a gargle, 85
Rous, Adam, Bequests of property to Prior and Convent of St Bartholomew, 9, 10, 19

Rous, Adam, Relations with (*a*) Johannes de Mirfeld, 9, 10, 19, 24, 34, 177; (*b*) John of Gaunt, 24; (*c*) Sir Robert de Swyllyngton, 15, 183
— — Surgeon to King Edward III, 3, 9, 24, 177

St John's College, Cambridge, MS. extracts of *Florarium* at, 170
Salerno, medical school of, 28, 29
Salerno, the School of, the Schola Salernitana, 29, 30, 43, 58, 59, 67, 73, 111, 112, 126, 127, 135, 137, 144–147, 152–155
Saliceto, William de, 105, 124, 125, 133
"Sanguis draconis" (dragon's-blood), an astringent medicine, 89
Schadelok, Margaret, 4, 8, 17, 176
Scruple, the, early use of, 93
Secret of Secrets, see *Secretum Secretorum*
Secretum Secretorum, 111, 112, 135–139, 144
Seneca, 130, 131
Sidonius Apollinaris, 130
"Signs of Death", *see De Signis Malis*
Simon of Sudbury (Bishop of London), 4, 17
Singer, Dr Charles, 70
Sinonoma, the (Glossary), 2, 37, 67, 81, 83, 84, 88, 89, 167
Sion College, London, 170, 173
Socrates, 144, 145
Solomon, King of Israel, 129, 159
Somer, John, astronomical calendar of, 38, 167
"Speculum", or "Mirror", the *Florarium* an example of, 54, 55, 103, 173
Sphere of Pythagoras, 70
"Spiritual healing", 108, 133
"Spiritual members", the, 81
"Spiritual physicians", *see* "Contra curatos"
Spodium, use of, as a medicine, 88
Sputum, in Phthisis, 75–79; *see also* Phlegm
Stomach, anatomy of, 151
Sugar of roses, efficacious in Phthisis, 83

Surgery, Clerks in Higher Orders forbidden to practise, 110, 129
Suthewelle, John de, 99–103, 115
Sutton, Elias de, 9, 13, 177, 178, 181
Swyllyngton, Sir Robert de (Kt), 15, 16, 182, 183
Sylvester, Bernard (of Chartres), 130
Syon Monastery, Isleworth, 170
Syrus, Publilius, 126

"Temperament", the, 32
"Thirteen pounds: Three years", story of dying Physician, 103, 131
Tortoise, bath prepared from, 87
Troy Weight, use of, 93
Twyne, Brian, 20, 21, 167
Tyngewich, Nicholas (Physician to Edward I and Professor of Medicine at Oxford), 21, 22, 110
Tyriac, 84, 85, 149

Ulceration of lung in Phthisis, 75, 79
Unction, Extreme, 108
"Unguentum Ptisicorum", 86, 87
Urine, use of, in prognosis, 67, 69

Vegetables, use of, in Phthisis, 83–85

"Versifier" (the unknown author of School of Salerno), 126, 127, 135–137, 153–155; see also Salerno, the School of
Vervain, use of, in prognosis, 67
Vincent of Beauvais, 131
"Vis Medicatrix Naturae", 125
Vomit, black, a sign of death, 61, 65
Vulgate, the, quotations from, 119, 121, 122, 127, 128, 134, 159, 161, 163
Vyne, William atte, woolmonger of London, 9, 10, 14, 177–179

Walter de Elvesden, his astronomical calendar, 37
Wat Tyler, 3
Webb, E. A., 3, 17
Weights and Measures, medical, 45, 92, 93, 167
William atte Vyne, see Vyne, William atte
Wine, beneficial for consumptives, 81
— its general and moderate use recommended, 147–149
Women doctors, indictment of, 122, 123
Worms, intestinal, as prognostic sign, 61
Wycliffe, John, 104, 133